MW00928617

*Discovering the*
# Word of Wisdom

# Praise for *Discovering the Word of Wisdom*

"The importance of diet is so fundamental to human survival and success that many of the world's religions have strongly encouraged their followers to eat a near vegan diet. Dr. Jane Birch has made an important contribution by retelling the truths about nutrition found in the Word of Wisdom in modern day language relevant to the reader."

— John A. McDougall, MD, author and founder of the McDougall Program

"There is so much confusion in the world today about what constitutes a healthy diet. As Latter-day Saints, we have a most valuable tool in the Word of Wisdom to help guide our dietary choices for optimal health, yet we succumb to the same chronic diseases as the rest of the civilized world. This book is a must read for anyone who wants to fully realize all the promised blessings found in the Word of Wisdom."

— Debra Christofferson, Registered Dietician; Research Professor of Nutrition, Utah State University

"Jane Birch's *Discovering the Word of Wisdom* combines scholarly research, personal stories, and gospel insights to create one of the most personally motivating books you will ever read about health. Her tone is positive and enlightening, and her work demonstrates the power of the Word of Wisdom to heal us, physically and spiritually."

— Christopher Foster, PhD; Professor of Philosophy; Founder of Mormons for Animals

"Jane Birch has written a much needed study of the broad implications of the Word of Wisdom for today. It will change the way you think and, more importantly, the way you consume. It gives new reason to believe in the inspiration of the prophet Joseph Smith."

— George Handley, PhD; Professor of Comparative Arts and Letters, Brigham Young University

"When I eat the way Jane suggests, I feel better. What greater evidence could there be?"

— Laura C. Bridgewater, PhD; Professor of Microbiology and Molecular Biology, Brigham Young University

"Through exuberant prose, Jane Birch carries us into the Eden possible through Word of Wisdom observance. Her book persuades the reader to reconsider lifetime habits of self-destruction and to replace them with habits of being in alignment with our divine nature."
— Dorothy A. Solomon, Dixie State University, author

"Jane Birch provides us with a much-needed reexamination of the Word of Wisdom in light of recent scientific research and continuing revelation. This is a fascinating study of how the Word of Wisdom has been interpreted over time and what meaning and value it has in a modern world of complex food choices. The reader is rewarded with fresh insights and much food for thought. This book provides a practical roadmap for using the Word of Wisdom to live a healthier, more productive, and spiritually fulfilling life."
— J. Michael Hunter, Mormon Studies Librarian, Harold B. Lee Library, Brigham Young University

"*Discovering the Word of Wisdom* captivated me! I feel energized by the possibilities of this healthy lifestyle. I'm confident all who read this book will learn something new. Want to feel better? Eat better! But watch out, Jane's enthusiasm for eating a plant-based diet is catching."
— Barbara M. Smith, Professor of Counseling Psychology and Special Education, Brigham Young University

"I have greatly appreciated reading this book by Jane Birch and the perspective she brings to the Word of Wisdom. . . . the closer we stick to the full perspective of D&C 89, the better we will feel physically and spiritually."
— Tim W. McGaughy, MD, PhD

"Hands down the best book I have ever read on the Word of Wisdom. It took me years and years of searching and seeking to find the information this ONE book so eloquently offers. You will feel enlightened, inspired, and have a deeper conviction toward better health from almost the moment you begin reading. In a world sinking deeper into confusion about health and nutrition, Jane offers the reader a source of utter clarity."
— Charity Lighten, Food for Life cooking instructor for The Cancer Project; co-founder, wholefoodmommies.com

"When I follow a whole food, plant-based diet I feel better—when I don't, I feel worse. It's that simple. Try it for yourself. As stated in Alma 32:27, 'awake and arouse your faculties, even to an experiment upon my words,' and see how it affects your health."
— Paul Caldarella, PhD; Associate Professor and Licensed Psychologist, Brigham Young University

"Jane asks many questions in her excellent book—'In a world of such confusion regarding healthful eating, *who can we trust?* Why are we as LDS not a healthier people?' With every question, she goes back to the Word of Wisdom for clarity, and offers fascinating historical and contemporary insights to help further elucidate this amazing revelation as she outlines the ideal diet for all of us. I cannot recommend this book highly enough. It is a must-read for anyone concerned about health—and even more so for anyone *not* concerned about health."
— Mavis Parkinson, MA, Theatre, Brigham Young University; Board of Governors, Utah Shakespeare Festival

"Jane's answer to a question she did not ask regarding a heart-attack proof diet should be a wake-up call for everyone consuming a typical American diet."
— Meldon K. Larson, MPA; Certified Internal Auditor, Brigham Young University

"Through careful research of the scientific literature and statements of past and present prophets, Jane Birch brings a unique perspective on a subject that is critically important in our time of increasing health challenges. She links the Word of Wisdom to the well-known work of such pillars of plant-based nutrition as Drs. Colin Campbell, Joel Fuhrman, John McDougall, and Caldwell Esselstyn, and demonstrates that the Word of Wisdom was, indeed, revealed for our day. Any serious scholar of nutrition and the Word of Wisdom must read Jane's seminal work."
— Julene Humes, Waldorf Early Child Educator; Director, Abella Cottage School

"*Discovering the Word of Wisdom* issues a provocative and personal invitation, built on scripture and science, to a healthier life."
— David H. Moore, JD; Professor of Law, Brigham Young University

"Dr. Jane Birch spoke to my sensibilities—indeed, to both my heart and mind—as never before in her book. As a decades-long member of the LDS Church, I supposed I understood the Word of Wisdom about as well as anyone. Yet the notion of the term 'sparingly' in reference to our use of animals came into clearer focus, thanks in part to Hugh Nibley's stunning interpretation, and in part to Jane's soul-provoking observation that 'ceasing enmity toward animals will lead to a greater depth of spirituality, sensitivity, and charity in the hearts of the Latter-day Saints and help prepare the earth for the Millennium.' I do not exaggerate in my claim that reading this book will change your life, if you so allow."
— Susan C. Eliason, Teaching and Learning Consultant, Center for Teaching and Learning, Brigham Young University

"Jane has summarized so many of the key principles I have found to be most effective in promoting my own health. When I follow these principles, I have more energy, less pressure from doctors, and peace of mind."
— David D. Williams, PhD; Professor of Instructional Psychology and Technology, Brigham Young University

"Reading this book will make you feel like you're talking to a trusted advisor as Jane poses and answers questions about the connection between a whole food, plant-based diet and an 1833 revelation that has never held more relevance to the health and vitality of the Saints than it does today. The real stories from LDS people living the Word of Wisdom are gems of personal inspiration that will speak to your heart and move you to action as people from all walks of life describe their experiences of awakening to the Word of Wisdom."
— Jessica Duffett, Speech-Language Pathologist, EdD candidate

"I love *Discovering the Word of Wisdom*! Jane Birch has compiled treasures of knowledge and truth into a format that is easy to read and speaks to my heart. She presents compelling evidence from revelation and science that we can find health and vitality by eating a whole food, plant-based diet. This book is an incredible resource for anyone who wants to receive a full measure of the blessings promised in the Word of Wisdom."
— Rebekah George, MPA; homemaker and mother of three

"I've read a few other books that compare and contrast the Standard American Diet with the Word of Wisdom. Jane's tops them all, because she combines scientific findings, words of ancient and modern prophets, her own personal journey, as well as other true healing experiences. Like many others, I spent years seeking for inspiration and searching out science that Jane synthesizes succinctly and simply in this short book. Many books and studies she cites are interesting but pretty difficult to read. Jane's *Discovering the Word of Wisdom* is better, because it is written without hype or excess jargon. Instead of confusion from designing men, Jane gives gospel clarity."
— Ginger Conrad, homemaker and healthy human

"Jane Birch is a living example of commitment to a challenging dietary lifestyle. Her book is a guide to the path of healthy eating and a testimony of the journey's blessings. A Zion people will live this way!"
— Joyce Kinmont, Founder of LDS Home Education Assn.; author of *Diet Decisions for Latter-day Saints*, ldsdietandhealth.org

"Jane's decision to make this radical life change occurred while I was working with her at BYU, and her gung-ho enthusiasm inspired me and my husband to examine our own eating habits. Ultimately we decided to take the plunge and noticed an incredible difference in the energy and health that ensued. The Word of Wisdom means so much more to us now that we live the do's just as much as we heed the don't's."
— Robyn Rowley, BS, Psychology, Brigham Young University

"What a gift Jane's book is to all people who are trying to live a quality, healthy lifestyle!"
— Tom and Carol Cherry, owners of Provo Piano Academy

"Jane Birch has a mission—an awakening to the real principles in the Word of Wisdom—so that we really shall run and not be weary, and walk and not faint."
— Stan and Sharon Miller, authors of *Especially for Mormons*; Provo Freedom Festival volunteers (27 years); Humanitarian Country Directors in the Hungary Budapest Mission

# Discovering the
# Word of Wisdom

## Surprising Insights from a
## Whole Food, Plant-based Perspective

℘

## Jane Birch

Fresh Awakenings
Provo, Utah

Copyright © 2013 by Abbie Jane Birch

All rights reserved. No portion of this book may be reproduced by any means without written permission from the author, except for quotations in reviews and non-profit educational purposes.

Fresh Awakenings
3172 Shadowbrook Circle
Provo, Utah, 84604

For more information or to purchase books:
discoveringthewordofwisdom.com
Order books toll free: 1-800-931-5960

ISBN-13: 978-1-4936849-6-0
ISBN-10: 1-4936849-6-5
First printing: November 2013
10 9 8 7 6 5 4 3 2

This book is not a publication of The Church of Jesus Christ of Latter-day Saints. All material herein is the responsibility of the author.

This book is not intended for individualized medical advice. Persons with medical conditions or who are taking medication should discuss any diet and lifestyle changes with their health professional.

Cover artwork by Clifford Lamb
Cover design by Bronson Terry
Typeset by Dustin Schwanger

This book is dedicated to my parents—
*J. Neil Birch and Judith Ann Birch*
They were the first to teach me the Word of Wisdom,
and they have been my biggest champions as I've adopted
a whole food, plant-based lifestyle.

With gratitude to my uncle—
*Clifford E. K. Lamb (1950-2010)*
He loved the Word of Wisdom. He taught us how to eat—
to praise God and care for our bodies. He was my angel in
writing this book, and his artwork adorns the cover.

*When health is absent, wisdom cannot reveal itself,*
*art cannot manifest, strength cannot fight, wealth becomes useless,*
*and intelligence cannot be applied.* — Herophilos (335–280 BC)

*And [they] shall find wisdom and great treasures of knowledge,*
*even hidden treasures.* (D&C 89:19)

*If you want to know what health is worth,*
*ask the person who has lost it.* — John Robbins (2001)

*[They] shall run and not be weary,*
*and shall walk and not faint.* (D&C 89:20)

# Contents

# Foreword

I grew up in the 1960's, and I can still remember the television commercials for cigarettes. I remember seeing the man on the horse in the great outdoors, smoking and promoting his brand. It wasn't long after viewing those ads that the science proving smoking is bad for us resulted in cigarette commercials being banned. As a child, I would read the Word of Wisdom, and I remember thinking, "Wow, the Word of Wisdom taught these principles almost 150 years ago, and now science is just figuring it out." Over the last 20 years, as I've studied diet and diet-related research, I've come to believe that the Word Wisdom goes beyond warning us against addictive substances—giving us knowledge, for example, that it is pleasing to God that we do not eat animals unless it is necessary. This too is now being confirmed by science.

My mother was the first person who introduced me to the idea that eating a meal without a meat entrée was okay. She made a wonderful garden skillet full of vegetables, and then served us a small handful of almonds as a side dish. We loved it! I also have a memory of my bishop and his family being vegetarians, though I thought maybe this was a little extreme. But not long after, when I was married and started studying medical research, I came across a study that linked red meat to breast cancer. I remember talking with my wife and suggesting to her that we probably should stop eating beef to avoid any chance of her developing breast cancer. Even though both our grandfathers were cattle ranchers, that did not deter us from making changes to our diet.

I became more interested in nutrition and tried to read everything related to diet. I soon came to know that eating animals or animal products was not healthy. In 1990, after reading some of the writings of Dr. John McDougall, I went to my wife and told her that I thought we should completely eliminate any meat and dairy products in our diet. She was a little skeptical at first, but as I explained the reasons, she agreed and was willing to give it a try. Our four children were young at the time. They seemed okay with the change, although initially we did have a little resistance from our oldest daughter, who was about 11 years old at that time. But within a few months, she too was committed. A couple of years later, we had our fifth child who was raised without ever eating meat, except when her so-called friends would try to trick her. (It's interesting that she is the tallest of our daughters.)

The result of this diet change had a profound impact on my health in very specific ways. Most of my life I had terrible allergies that seemed to flare up in the spring and summer with the pollen and dried weeds. I coughed and sneezed and had watery eyes. I wanted to take a wire brush to the back of my throat. I also occasionally experienced what I thought was exercise-induced asthma that seemed to be related to the allergy flare-ups. Then we changed our diet. That was in November and after the next summer came and went, I realized I had not had one allergy flare-up, and I have never had one since. I consider this a great blessing in my life and know it is a blessing of more fully living the Word Wisdom

In my professional life as a physical therapist I have continued to read and study everything I can on diet. In 2010 I completed the Plant-based Nutrition Certificate program from eCornell. I take every opportunity to talk to patients about their diet and encourage all to study for themselves the current literature and learn so that they can make the best decision for their own health. Colin Campbell's book, *The China Study*, has been an important tool in teaching and helping people make healthy changes. I have sold (at cost) 48 cases (over 1,500 books) of *The China Study* since 2005. It has been exciting for me to watch patients and friends as they learn scientific facts, and as they begin to understand the Word of Wisdom more clearly. As they make positive changes, they see their health improve dramatically.

I have noticed there are two kinds of people who are willing to change their diet. First are those who learn the truth and follow it. The second are those who are challenged with a health crisis and are compelled to seek further understanding and help. I would recommend being among the former rather than the latter. As we learn the scientific facts, we begin to understand the Word of Wisdom more clearly. When science lines up with scripture, we have added confirmation that we have found the truth.

When I first read Dr. Jane Birch's story of her conversion to a plant-based diet, I was surprised that in such a short time she had thoroughly researched and discovered the scientific knowledge and the insights the scriptures provide related to diet. She has a phenomenal hunger for knowledge, which has served her well in researching the Word of Wisdom and its relationship to the current body of scientific knowledge that can direct all of us to a healthier lifestyle. In her book *Discovering the Word of Wisdom: Surprising Insights from a Whole Food, Plant-based Perspective*, she provides real stories of individuals whose lives have been changed, giving further evidence of the profound effect the things we eat have on our health. These stories are powerful examples of the promised blessings given to those who have the courage to change their lives to embrace aspects of the Word of Wisdom that may not align with the standard American diet.

I believe the Word of Wisdom is a gift from our Heavenly Father. I believe every verse in the Word of Wisdom with all my heart. What a magnificent section of scripture—diet-related direction provided by God in a world so fraught with confusion. I believe Jane's insights into the Word of Wisdom can provide readers with a wealth of knowledge and understanding that can impact their lives with health and the promised "wisdom and great treasures of knowledge" (D&C 89:19). Her book is a gift to us. As we gain a greater understanding of the Word of Wisdom, and do everything within our power to align our lives with it, we will receive the promised blessings.

Rogan Taylor, DPT
Spine, Orthopedic & Sports Physical Therapy
Provo, Utah
September 19, 2013

# Preface

I never imagined I'd feel this passionate about diet, nutrition, and preventing chronic disease. Considering how important the topic is, and how much research has gone into investigating it, you'd think by now we'd know all the answers. What could possibly be left to get excited about? Before writing this book, I knew little about the strongly held, diverse opinions currently thriving in the marketplace of ideas on diet and nutrition. Now that I've spent years studying the wide variety of educated opinions, I am convinced our society will never come to a consensus for what constitutes the optimal human diet.

Anyone who delves into the nutritional debates might well feel something akin to what Joseph Smith, the founder of The Church of Jesus Christ of Latter-day Saints, felt in the midst of the "war of words and tumult of opinions" of various religious denominations. He wrote:

> So great were the confusion and strife . . . that it was impossible for a person young as I was, and so unacquainted with men and things, to come to any certain conclusion who was right and who was wrong. . . . I often said to myself: What is to be done? Who of all these parties are right; or, are they all wrong together? (Joseph Smith—History 1:8, 10)

Today we are in the midst of a "war of words and tumult of opinions" on what we should eat. How are we to decide what is right? Fortunately, we have a revelation from God in modern-day scripture: Doctrine and Covenants (D&C) Section 89, which we call the "Word of Wisdom." We can also pray to God, as Joseph did. But we generally do not realize how much our lack of knowledge, personal preferences, and cultural traditions impact our understanding of this revelation and make it difficult to receive unambiguous communication from the Lord. Just as the Word of Wisdom helps us evaluate the nutritional opinions of our day, so do the nutritional opinions of our day color our interpretation of the Word of Wisdom, as well as the way we hear the Lord's counsel to us as individuals.

I have heard the Word of Wisdom used to justify all types of contradictory nutritional advice. It is clear that what D&C 89 tells us is not completely unambiguous, beyond what LDS Church leaders have made plain. It certainly was not clear to me. All of that changed one fateful day when I heard a few ideas about nutrition expressed so plainly and so convincingly I knew those ideas were true and that my life would never be the same again. Surprisingly, it wasn't until sometime later that I realized these same truths were contained within a revelation I was very familiar with: the Word of Wisdom.

An LDS Article of Faith proclaims, "We believe [God] will yet reveal many great and important things pertaining to the Kingdom of God" (Article 9). In the past when I pictured this article of faith coming to pass, I envisioned rather dramatic unveilings: a special session of General Conference where the Prophet announces new, spectacular revelations straight from God; the opening of the sealed portions of the Book of Mormon; or the Lost Tribes showing up in Salt Lake City with their scriptures. What I did not imagine was that some of the "great and important things" to be revealed might already be contained in the same set of scriptures I've had my entire life, just waiting for me to finally catch a glimpse of what they mean. This is how I now feel about the Word of Wisdom.

The interesting fact in my story is that it took people who are not members of the LDS Church, who know nothing about the Word of Wisdom, to help me discover a whole new way of thinking about the verses in Section 89. What I have learned has been not just mind expanding, but also soul expanding. While the unfolding of this revelation to my mind has not been a public event, it has in every other sense been a dramatic unveiling of new and spectacular revelations containing "many great and important things pertaining to the Kingdom of God."

Just as importantly, as my mind has opened up to a deeper understanding of the Word of Wisdom, so has this understanding opened my mind to better evaluate the wisdom of the world. It has also given me courage. In my study of nutrition, I've encountered several key crossroads where I have wondered whether I'm on the right path, or where I have doubted whether there is a right path and whether it is possible to know it. Time after time, I have found it helpful to return to the Word of Wisdom. It has become the anchor of my study, the measure by which I can evaluate the "tumult of opinions" and scientific "facts" in the marketplace of ideas.

This book is about discovering the words of wisdom contained in D&C 89. Most of the ideas in this book will resonate with the majority of readers who are members of the LDS Church because of their familiarity with the Word of Wisdom. I also hope it will appeal to those not of this faith. I expect that a great many of the ideas presented in this book will be new to readers, as they were to me. From the responses I've received from initial readers, these concepts are not only new, but valuable and potentially life changing. I share them with humility and a sincere desire to bless others with ideas that have been revolutionary in my life. I believe they can be revolutionary in your life as well.

In many ways, it is a bold (and maybe foolish) attempt to write about the Word of Wisdom. Many Latter-day Saint authors have gone before me, and it is clear in hindsight that so much of what they passionately declared to be eternal truth was, in fact, heavily colored by the science of their day and is now quite dated. I know this book is also not a perfect work, but I believe the message it contains is too important to wait until the book is perfect before publishing it. I also feel readers need not wait for it to be perfected before they benefit from the ideas it contains.

I hope you will read this book and then read, study, and ponder again the words in the Word of Wisdom. Ask God to guide you. He has given us the Word of Wisdom for a reason. The evolution of our collective understanding of what He revealed in 1833 has been a long and gradual process that continues to unfold in our day. I am now convinced that at least some of the "great and important things" God will "yet reveal" to us are contained in D&C 89, the section where God has given us precious words of wisdom on what, why, and how we should consume the foods He has ordained for our use. I hope this book can be a turning point for interested members of the Church (and those not of this faith) in their discovery and practice of the Word of Wisdom.

All profits from the sale of this book (should there be any sales!) will go toward making more resources freely available to whoever would like more information (you can sign up at discoveringthewordofwisdom.com).

# A Brief Explanation of the Word of Wisdom

The "Word of Wisdom" refers to a revelation Mormons believe God gave through Joseph Smith, Jr., the founder of The Church of Jesus Christ of Latter-day Saints, in 1833. In this revelation, God explains what is and is not ordained for human consumption. The text of the Word of Wisdom is rich and includes many dimensions, but the dietary advice might be summarized as follows:

1. Strong drinks (alcohol), tobacco, and "hot drinks" (defined later as "coffee and tea") should not be consumed.
2. All wholesome plants are ordained for human use.
3. Meat is ordained for human use, but it should be eaten sparingly and only in times of winter, cold, famine or "excess of hunger."
4. All grain is good and is ordained to be the staff of life.

The Word of Wisdom promises rich blessings to those who keep these sayings, along with the other commandments of God.

This revelation can be found, along with many other revelations Joseph Smith received, in a book Mormons believe is latter-day scripture: the *Doctrine and Covenants* (D&C). The Word of Wisdom is the 89th revelation contained in that book, so the text is also commonly referred to as Doctrine and Covenants 89, D&C 89 or simply Section 89. The full text is printed below.

# Doctrine and Covenants Section 89

1 A Word of Wisdom, for the benefit of the council of high priests, assembled in Kirtland, and the church, and also the saints in Zion—

2 To be sent greeting; not by commandment or constraint, but by revelation and the word of wisdom, showing forth the order and will of God in the temporal salvation of all saints in the last days—

3 Given for a principle with promise, adapted to the capacity of the weak and the weakest of all saints, who are or can be called saints.

4 Behold, verily, thus saith the Lord unto you: In consequence of evils and designs which do and will exist in the hearts of conspiring men in the last days, I have warned you, and forewarn you, by giving unto you this word of wisdom by revelation—

5 That inasmuch as any man drinketh wine or strong drink among you, behold it is not good, neither meet in the sight of your Father, only in assembling yourselves together to offer up your sacraments before him.

6 And, behold, this should be wine, yea, pure wine of the grape of the vine, of your own make.

7 And, again, strong drinks are not for the belly, but for the washing of your bodies.

8 And again, tobacco is not for the body, neither for the belly, and is not good for man, but is an herb for bruises and all sick cattle, to be used with judgment and skill.

9 And again, hot drinks are not for the body or belly.

10 And again, verily I say unto you, all wholesome herbs God hath ordained for the constitution, nature, and use of man—

11 Every herb in the season thereof, and every fruit in the season thereof; all these to be used with prudence and thanksgiving.

12 Yea, flesh also of beasts and of the fowls of the air, I, the Lord, have ordained for the use of man with thanksgiving; nevertheless they are to be used sparingly;

13 And it is pleasing unto me that they should not be used, only in times of winter, or of cold, or famine.

14 All grain is ordained for the use of man and of beasts, to be the staff of life, not only for man but for the beasts of the field, and the fowls of heaven, and all wild animals that run or creep on the earth;

15 And these hath God made for the use of man only in times of famine and excess of hunger.

16 All grain is good for the food of man; as also the fruit of the vine; that which yieldeth fruit, whether in the ground or above the ground—

17 Nevertheless, wheat for man, and corn for the ox, and oats for the horse, and rye for the fowls and for swine, and for all beasts of the field, and barley for all useful animals, and for mild drinks, as also other grain.

18 And all saints who remember to keep and do these sayings, walking in obedience to the commandments, shall receive health in their navel and marrow to their bones;

19 And shall find wisdom and great treasures of knowledge, even hidden treasures;

20 And shall run and not be weary, and shall walk and not faint.

21 And I, the Lord, give unto them a promise, that the destroying angel shall pass by them, as the children of Israel, and not slay them. Amen.

# 1

# Awakening to the Word of Wisdom

I'd always pitied vegetarians. Vegans were beyond comprehension. It would be awful enough to give up meat, but why would anyone give up butter, cheese—or worse, *ice cream?!* Is life worth living without feta cheese or Rocky Road? So, imagine my surprise when on August 20, 2011, I suddenly became so convinced of the health hazards of eating animal foods that I gave them up completely, with no thought (not even a desire) of eating them again.

Several months later I was chatting with my nephew, Christian Lloyd. He began eating a vegetarian diet as a young teen (and yes, I had pitied him). He asked me, "Before you stopped eating meat, what did you think of those verses in the Word of Wisdom?" I knew exactly which verses he meant:

> Yea, flesh also of beasts and of the fowls of the air, I, the Lord, have ordained for the use of man with thanksgiving; nevertheless they are to be used sparingly; And it is pleasing unto me that they should not be used, only in times of winter, or of cold, or famine. (D&C 89:12–13)

It was true that as many times as I had read these verses, they had failed to impact how I ate. Nevertheless I told my nephew, "I thought the same way I think now: these verses seem clear and unambiguous—why doesn't anyone talk about them?"

## My Longing to "Run and Not Be Weary"

I've always loved the Word of Wisdom, but its promised blessings became particularly meaningful to me after I began experiencing severe, sometimes crippling pain in my legs in the year 2000. I prayed long and hard to find an answer. I went to every type of medical and alternative health specialist I could find. During the years that followed, I sometimes felt better, but the pain never went away. How I longed for the blessing promised in the Word of Wisdom to "run and not be weary" and "walk and not faint" (D&C 89:20). In fact, this particular phrase went through my mind over and over again during long years of wondering if I'd ever walk freely again.

I decided to devote the summer of 2011 to finding a solution to the pain in my legs. I ended up seeing several medical specialists, and on July 20, 2011, I finally got my answer. On that day I learned I have a congenital condition called *developmental dysplasia of the hip*. I was told, in no uncertain terms, that the only solution was major hip surgery.

I had no idea I'd be so unhappy to get my answer. I would have done anything, short of surgery, to try to correct the problem. I was willing to follow any type of diet, physical therapy, meditation, or exercise (even yoga!). I didn't want to believe that none of these solutions addressed my problem, nor did I want to feel stuck with an answer that made me very unhappy. There was just no way I was going to have surgery!

Once I got the diagnosis, my life was consumed with coming to grips with what I was learning. My effort to find an answer so occupied my attention that I spent little time thinking of anything else.

## An Answer to a Question I Did Not Ask

Exactly one month to the day after being diagnosed, I suddenly received an answer to a question I did not ask, one that was not even on my radar screen. It was Saturday, August 20, 2011. I woke up much earlier than usual and went into the living room where my good friend, Abbie Kim, had the TV on and tuned to CNN. If she hadn't been there that morning, I would never have seen the preview for a program Dr. Sanjay Gupta was doing called "The Last Heart Attack."

A few moments into this preview, I learned that Dr. Gupta was investigating a "heart-attack proof" diet, which sounded very strange to me. At first I thought he'd be debunking some quack idea because it seemed impossible that a person could become literally "heart-attack proof," but after watching the preview I realized Dr. Gupta was serious. Based on his research, he asserted there is a diet that can prevent heart disease. This was interesting to me, not because I had any risk factors for heart disease, but because I'd often heard it is the number one killer in America, that one out of every two men and one out of every three women will suffer from heart disease. What if we could eliminate heart disease in America through diet? What would that save us in money, in suffering, and premature death? This grabbed my attention. It was still very early on a Saturday morning, but I was now wide awake.

After a big breakfast that totally contradicted the advice Dr. Gupta had just shared, I started researching the diet on the Internet, beginning with the doctor featured in the CNN preview, Dr. Caldwell Esselstyn of the Cleveland Clinic. I quickly found plenty of solid information and was surprised that it looked much more compelling than I had expected. I was especially impressed that (just as the CNN preview suggested) there appeared to be specific and reliable scientific and clinical evidence that the featured diet doesn't just *reduce* our chance of getting heart disease, but actually *eliminates* it. This impressed me. It is not easy to make big changes, and I do not feel very motivated to make dramatic lifestyle changes when it only *reduces* my chances of having problems; it feels like a gamble. *Eliminating* my chance of getting a disease, especially the number one killer, felt very motivating to me.

Equally important, I soon learned that the recommended diet does much more than make us "heart-attack proof." I was astounded to learn that by eating a "heart-attack proof" diet, I could also drastically reduce or (in many cases) eliminate my chance of ever having to deal with most of the other chronic problems common on our society:

| | | |
|---|---|---|
| Arthritis (AS, gout, psoriatic, rheumatoid) | Diabetes | Hypertension |
| Atherosclerosis (heart disease, carotid artery disease, strokes) | Diverticulitis | Kidney disease |
| Asthma | Erectile dysfunction | Kidney stones |
| Cancers (colon, breast, uterus, ovary, kidney, prostate) | Gallstones | Multiple sclerosis |
| Cataracts & macular degeneration | Gastritis (ulcers) | Obesity |
| Colitis (Crohn's, ulcerative) | Hearing loss | Osteoporosis |
| Constipation | Hemorrhoids | Parkinson's disease |
| Dementia (Alzheimer's, cognitive dysfunction) | Hiatus hernia | Varicose veins |

Up to this point in my life, I hadn't thought much about becoming chronically ill; I just assumed we'd all end up with one or more of these diseases during our lifetimes, especially as we get older. I hadn't spent much time worrying about them since eventual poor health seemed inevitable. I figured I'd "cross that bridge" when I got there. But now the thought of living my life with a dramatically reduced chance of ever getting any of these diseases sounded pretty good. I started to consider what type of lifestyle change would NOT be worth these results. I started to think about what good health is worth to me. I thought about a very prominent, extremely wealthy man in our community who suffered from diabetes and heart disease. With all the money and power he had, he was not able to save his legs from amputation, or then even his own life, though he suffered from chronic diseases that could have been prevented through diet. He was just 64 years old.

Of course I was interested in exactly what the diet included and excluded. I learned it is called a "whole food, plant-based" (WFPB) diet. "Whole food" means very limited or no processed foods (including refined oils). "Plant-based" means meals based on plant rather than animal foods (which include meat, dairy, and eggs). What it includes are four food groups: unprocessed vegetables, fruits, legumes (beans, peas and lentils), and whole grains. In other words, *whole plants*, packaged as God (or nature) designed them.

The evidence backing how this diet leads to the results it claims was surprisingly convincing to me as I realized there is a direct link between the way we eat and how well our bodies function. Food is obviously the most intimate contact we have with our environment; we consume several pounds of food day in and day out. How could food not have a dramatic impact on our health?

I learned that Dr. Caldwell Esselstyn worked with patients with severe coronary artery disease, 100 percent of whom were able to stop or even reverse the progression of their disease when following this diet. Since his initial study, he has worked with hundreds of additional patients, all with the same results. Likewise, people following this same diet (whether under the care of a doctor or on their own) have successfully and consistently stopped and even reversed the progression of other diet-related chronic illnesses.

The combined evidence for this line of thinking, from even my brief study that Saturday morning, had an unpredictable effect on me. Within a relatively short amount of time (less than a few hours after watching the

CNN preview), I came to the astonishing conclusion that, based on my evaluation of the evidence, I had better change my entire way of eating. For lunch that same day I began eating a WFPB diet. My first meal? Fresh corn on the cob *sans* butter. It was delicious, even without the extra fat. I was overjoyed. I was off to a great start!

## Learning to Live with a New Diet

In my excitement over discovering new truths, it took a little time to realize what a radical effect this dietary change would have on my daily life. What I had not considered was my total lack of culinary skills. If I didn't even know how to cook "normal" food, how could I ever cook this strange stuff?! Being single and not having to cook for a family had made it easy for me (as it is for most Americans) to get by on convenient, readily available foods. The few foods I did make were quick and easy and tasted good because our modern food culture makes this incredibly simple.

All this changed dramatically with my new diet. I slowly realized that if I stuck to the diet, my food consumption from here on out would be entirely my own responsibility. Before this, I confess I occasionally sponged off of kind souls who were more than willing to feed me. But no one I knew cooked like this, and we certainly don't have many WFPB restaurants in Utah County! Now, I'd have to prepare nearly everything I ate, and I couldn't rely on the easy shortcuts our society has created to make yummy food creation a painless process. Without the refined foods, sugars, and fats of my past diet, figuring out how to make "whole food" taste good soon became a big challenge. Fortunately, I felt so committed to giving this my best try that even days of eating far-less-than-yummy foods did not make me want to give up.

During the next few weeks, I definitely was NOT enjoying my new diet. People who had been eating this way for years told me that my taste buds would change. I tried to imagine I could learn to cook. I tried not to think about food tasting like this for the rest of my life and instead focused on getting through the next few months while I figured things out.

Through reading online forums, I got to know some of the many people who eat this way. I discovered they truly enjoy their food and are experiencing the promised weight loss and increased energy and good health. In reading their stories, I couldn't doubt their sincerity. Their food tastes had changed. It was obvious they relished their new foods with the same joy I had always gotten from eating. And, without all the added fat, sugar, and processed foods, they felt they could (for the first time) truly savor the subtle, delicious flavors of whole plant foods. They also appreciated a diet that did not make them count calories or stop eating before they were full. With this diet, you can eat as much as you need (to satiety), never go hungry, and still lose excess weight.

I quickly found hundreds of recipes to support this diet. I tried many. They all failed. While others loved the food, I did not. I was now eating food to stay alive but not for enjoyment or pleasure. I did feel great after every meal, never weighed down or heavy. I had energy, and I felt strong and healthy. I was losing weight. But I was discouraged. I was committed to the diet, but I wanted it to be easy, and it was not.[1]

## The Evidence Mounts, and I Share My Enthusiasm

Over the next few weeks, I continued to study the new diet. The first book I read was *The China Study* by T. Colin Campbell.[2] In this tour de force on nutrition and diet, Campbell presents not only the "most comprehensive study of nutrition ever conducted," but also the results of hundreds of other mainstream scientific studies, all with the same compelling conclusion: the unquestionable benefits of a whole food, plant-based diet. It didn't take even a full chapter to convince me. I was sold.

The more I researched, the more impressed I became. This excitement is unusual for me. We all hear about "miracle" cures, wonder nutrients, and super foods. I've been tempted to get excited about a few of the pitches, but I have always listened with a grain of salt, knowing that most such miracles do not work better than placebos and are not backed by solid science. Others work for some but not for everyone. Most contradict each other and make the whole subject of health and nutrition confusing and discouraging.

We've all heard from people who are overly passionate about this or that supplement or super food: acai berries, wheatgrass, cold-pressed coconut oil, probiotics, krill oil, CoQ10, etc. We are regularly bombarded with news of health-altering wonder nutrients, and I'm sure they all have their merits, but the WFPB diet felt very different. This struck me as transparently and unambiguously true. It was not gimmicky; it rang true to history, science, and common sense; no one stood to make money by converting me to it; and I couldn't help but notice it resonated with truths that were already an important part of who I am: the truths found in the Word of Wisdom.

Things began falling into place once I realized that as I used the principles of this diet as the large, foundational building blocks, all other nutrition facts finally began to make sense. In fact, learning these principles helped me better understand all competing claims and make sense out of the seeming confusion. I was beginning to see the forest for the trees. It was thrilling!

Like any new convert, I wanted to share what I was learning with others. I knew I had discovered hidden treasures—treasures "hidden" in plain sight. I became eager to let others know there are jewels lying all around us, enough for everyone to scoop up by the dozens. But these treasures are much more valuable than diamonds and pearls because they promise "health in their navel and marrow to their bones . . . wisdom and great treasures of knowledge, even hidden treasures" (D&C 89:19).

In my enthusiasm, I began a campaign to help friends, family, and colleagues at work learn about a whole food, plant-based diet. I wanted them to understand the basic principles before they or someone they loved experienced chronic illness. I hoped they'd feel even a part of the joy I was feeling as my understanding of diet and nutrition rapidly expanded. I shared my enthusiasm with everyone who would listen.

## Something Changes

For myself, somewhere between week seven and eight I suddenly realized I was enjoying my food! I can't be sure whether it was my taste buds changing or my cooking improving. Maybe it had just been so long since I had had lasagna or cheesecake that I forgot what "good" food tastes like. No matter. I began thoroughly enjoying three very large meals a day. I looked forward to eating; I ate with relish; and I felt fully satisfied after every meal. I had plenty of tasty whole food, plant-based snacks when I wanted them. I didn't count carbs or calories. I felt fantastic!

Other than the congenital hip condition, I didn't have any major health issues when I started the diet, but I did hope to lose weight. After high school I had gradually put on 45 pounds of unneeded weight (fat, not muscle!). In 2005, I started to cut back on calories to keep from ballooning out any further, and I very slowly began to lose weight. Over the next six years (between 2005 and the time I started this diet in 2011), I lost 20 pounds. After starting this diet, I lost 15 pounds in 12 weeks and 25 pounds in seven months (going from a BMI of 24 to 20). All without going hungry!

Of course, many others have started this diet much heavier and with serious, sometimes even chronic, diseases. The stories of how their health turned around dramatically in even a few short months are eye-opening and inspiring. My story is much less dramatic. I had my cholesterol tested at the three-month mark. My total cholesterol and LDL levels (originally 199 and 137) had both dropped 32 percent. My total cholesterol is now 130 and is in the "ideal" range (<150), a range that is common in populations where heart disease (and cancer) is nearly non-existent. When I had my carotid arteries checked in 2012, I was told they look like someone *half* my age. *All* of the small health issues I had also disappeared: a saliva gland that had been blocked for 10 years, annoyingly dry eyes, extremely itchy spots on my body, leg cramps at night, and occasional constipation. Since changing my diet, I feel great, enjoy plenty of energy, and am finally sleeping well.

Here is how I figure: I enjoyed *plenty* of meat and junk foods during the first half of my life. Now, I can enjoy different foods and better health the second half of my life. After all, what is health worth? And what have I really given up? I eat lots of delicious food, which I thoroughly enjoy. It is less expensive to buy and will save me in healthcare dollars in the future. In addition, I have the opportunity to share something precious with others, and maybe one day I'll have the privilege of making a difference in the health of another person. I have lost little and gained much.

I have thought a lot about why I made such a radical change that day in August. This diet was not an answer to a question I had. I had no known risk factors for any major illness. I was feeling healthy at the time, and I was eating as sensibly as (or more sensibly than) most people. God answered a prayer I did not give. But when I learned that by simply eating differently, I could prevent most of the chronic diseases so common in our society, I quickly decided that no amount of sacrifice in my diet was too dramatic. I had just endured more than a decade of pain; I knew what that had cost me in money, time, worry, social isolation, disability, and distress. I know we cannot avoid all suffering in this life—that is not part of God's plan. But since God had just given me an answer that promised dramatically better health, there was just no way that I was going to ignore it.

What I was not expecting when I made that decision was to discover that everything I was now learning about good health and nutrition was already contained in a document that was very familiar to me—Section 89 of the Doctrine and Covenants, the Word of Wisdom.

My primary task in this book is to explore how a whole food, plant-based diet helps us better understand the counsel given in D&C 89. In doing so, I'll present the scientific facts that seem clear and noncontroversial to me (though I know they are controversial to others). But I also need to explain that this book will not attempt to make the scientific argument for a whole food, plant-based diet. This has been done very well elsewhere. There is a substantial body of research, published in peer-reviewed journals, to support almost every scientific claim in this book. In my personal study, I *often* go to these original research articles to verify the claims of the experts I read. But because this body of literature is so vast and my primary goal is not to establish the *scientific* case, in this book I usually cite the secondary research of whole food, plant-based experts rather than the peer-reviewed literature itself. Interested readers can easily locate a substantial amount of primary research through the many citations in the books I reference. I encourage readers to make this a serious subject of investigation, should this interest them (see Appendix Seven, especially *The China Study*).

## Real Mormons ℘ Real Stories

### *Lynn's Story*

As a teenage boy I could eat anything and never put on a pound. However, as an adult, I found myself putting on weight until I weighed over 50 pounds more than I did in high school. My job as a BYU faculty member involved mostly sitting at a desk or standing in front of a class. That led to physical problems. At age 40, running and even walking produced pain in my knees that reduced my activity level even further. Nevertheless, I accepted this reduction and the accompanying gain in weight as part of the normal aging process. I didn't worry much about it. I exercised moderately and consumed a diet relatively high in refined flour, sugar, dairy products, and meat, which I had been taught were "good food."

When I was in my forties and fifties, a high school or college classmate or family member my age, who had been a healthy or even athletic youth, would occasionally appear in the obituaries—usually a victim of a heart attack, stroke, or cancer. Also, among those who were still alive, I noticed a significant number growing (in their own words) "slower, fatter, and stupider" and accepting these undesirable changes as inevitable.

In my early fifties, I started caring for my mother, who (like many people of her era) had never engaged in serious physical exercise or consumed very healthful food. She raised us on a standard American diet—white bread, hamburger, bologna, eggs, milk, and potatoes and gravy, with small side helpings of peas, green beans, or corn topped with butter. In fact, she slathered butter on nearly everything "to make it slip down your throat." It should come as no surprise that she had high cholesterol, high blood pressure, and low energy—especially as she entered her seventies. She just wanted to sit in her recliner and "save her strength." Over the ensuing years, she suffered a series of ministrokes (caused by clogged arteries to the brain). Her vascular dementia robbed her of her mental powers. One Christmas, she suffered a heart attack, which left her weak even after the cardiologists placed a stent in her clogged coronary artery. After that followed congestive heart failure, breast cancer, diabetes, and other diseases that did not kill her but robbed her of a meaningful life, wore out her husband, ravaged their hard-earned life savings, and exhausted her family caretakers, like me. She declined slowly and sadly over a decade.

Caring for my aging mother through her declining years was a hard but valuable life lesson for me. Sometimes, she would point her finger at me and say, "You just wait; your turn is coming!" as if what she was suffering in her old age was my unavoidable fate. I earnestly hoped she was wrong and vowed to do everything in my power to stay active and healthy as long as I could in order to remain independent and productive in my senior years and spare my family the pain and expense that come with an aging process so many modern Americans have come to accept as "normal."

When I was 53 years old, I enrolled in the "Y-Be-Fit" program at BYU and had my body and blood analyzed. I was shocked to find that my body was "obese" and that my cholesterol level (220) was in the "moderate risk" range. Even worse, when I started exercising more seriously, my cholesterol stubbornly remained at unhealthy levels, above 200. I started taking statin drugs, but my cholesterol level still stayed between 170 and 180, which was far from ideal and made me think that maybe my mother's grim prediction would come true.

Shortly after turning 60, I happened across a book titled *Younger Next Year* by Chris Crowley and Henry Lodge, MD. It explained that many of the leading causes of death in our modern Western society (heart disease, stroke, cancer) are attributable in large part to lifestyle. They cited research findings that determined that 70 percent of what we believe is normal aging is "optional." I decided it was time to change my lifestyle.

Soon thereafter, a friend in my ward, who teaches physical education at BYU, gave a lesson in our high priest group on the obesity epidemic in America and its astronomical financial, physical, and social costs to our society. This good colleague and brother also introduced me to *Forks Over Knives*, a video that explains the research of Dr. T. Colin Campbell and Dr. Caldwell B. Esselstyn, Jr., which concludes that a plant-based, whole foods diet can reduce or even prevent many of the lifestyle diseases that cause so much premature death, disease, and suffering in our society. I was attracted by the fit between the basic findings of Campbell's and Esselstyn's work and the positive aspects of the Word of Wisdom—the eating of grains, fruits, and vegetables in abundance and of meat sparingly (while not even mentioning milk and eggs as food sources).

About that time, I was at Costco one Saturday and watched a Vitamix demonstrator whip up a "green smoothie." It was delicious, not to mention healthy. We already had a Vitamix at home, so it was a simple thing to start using it to make tasty and healthy green and orange smoothies (from spinach, carrots, kale, apple, banana, pineapple, etc.), which I drank twice a day. At the same time, I cut way back on meat and dairy products and increased my consumption of whole grains and legumes. My wife's parents were immigrants from Japan, so she was pleased to add more Japanese-style vegetables to our meals.

When I changed my diet in these ways, an amazing thing happened. My weight, which had been so resistant to change, began to drop. Over a couple of months, I lost nearly 15 pounds, but when my weight reached the "ideal" (according to the charts) for my height and my BMI was right in the middle of the "normal" range (21), it stopped dropping. There it stayed for many months, as long as I stuck to my plant-based, whole foods diet. If I relaxed, however, and reverted to my old dietary habits, my weight would creep back up. For most of the past two years, I am pleased to report, it has stayed near "ideal."

Just as my weight dropped, so did my cholesterol levels. As mentioned, for nearly twenty years, my total cholesterol had been well above 200 (as high as 239) almost every time it was measured. Being in the "moderate risk" category wasn't very comforting. As I turned 50, however, my cholesterol level reached new heights (240-260), putting me in the "high risk" category. Statin drug therapy lowered my cholesterol, but it was still not ideal. When I switched to a plant-based diet, however, I finally reached my goal of "ideal" (<150) cholesterol levels. A recent blood test reported my cholesterol level is 130.

I can also report that since turning 60 I have had more energy and less disease than I did previously. Besides running for exercise, I started running for fun. At first, I ran 5K races, which were all I could manage. In 2012 (at age 62) I ran my first 10K race and surprised myself by winning the trophy for first place in my age category. In 2013, I ran a half marathon. And since turning 60, I have participated in three triathlons, winning a bronze, silver, or gold medal in my age category each time. That's not bad for someone who gave up running twenty years earlier because of knee pain! But I don't run to win medals. Although I am tired at the end of each of these races, I find a joyful sense of accomplishment in simply completing them. I see each success as a fulfillment of the promise of the Word of Wisdom that those who keep not only the "don't's" but also the "do's" of this counsel from God "shall run and not be weary, and shall walk and not faint" (D&C 89:20).

*Lynn Henrichsen, age 63, is a professor of Linguistics and English Language at Brigham Young University. He and his wife live in Provo, Utah. They have four children and ten grandchildren. He holds a doctorate degree in education and has studied eight foreign languages, worked in or visited 26 countries, and has taught students from over 60 different nations.*

Additional stories are included at the end of each chapter and in Appendix One: *More* Real Mormons ∾ Real Stories.

# 2

# The Flesh of Beasts

As I mentioned in the first chapter, in my eagerness to share my new diet with others, I told my story to anyone who would listen. I also explained to them the fundamentals of the diet: eating *whole* (not refined or heavily processed) *plant-based* (not animal) foods. This excludes much, if not all, meat, and one of the first questions I got when I shared the diet with others was, "But what about the Word of Wisdom?" The implication seemed to be, "Aren't we supposed to eat meat sparingly?" This line of questioning led me to ponder the words of Section 89 more carefully:

> Yea, flesh also of beasts and of the fowls of the air, I, the Lord, have ordained for the use of man with thanksgiving; nevertheless they are to be used sparingly. (D&C 89:12)

What might the instruction to eat meat "sparingly" mean? Here are some definitions of the word *sparingly* from the 1828 *Webster's Dictionary*:

1. Not abundantly.
2. Frugally; parsimoniously; not lavishly.
3. Abstinently; moderately.
4. Seldom; not frequently.
5. Cautiously; tenderly.[1]

Given these definitions, I realized that I had already consumed so much meat in the first 50 years of life that if I never ate another piece of meat for the next 50 years, the average amount of meat I'd have consumed by the end of my life could never, as a whole, be considered "sparingly"! But as helpful as verse 12 is in helping us understand the role of meat in the

Lord's diet plan, the next verse in Section 89 gives us further insight into the Lord's intent:

> And it is pleasing unto me that they should not be used, only in times of winter, or of cold, or famine. (D&C 89:13)

This is reiterated, perhaps even clarified, in verse 15:

> And these hath God made for the use of man only in times of famine and excess of hunger. (D&C 89:15)

The commonsense meaning of these verses is that we are asked to eat very little meat, and further that it "pleases the Lord" if we don't eat meat at all except in times of need, as in times of cold or famine when plant foods are scarce and our survival may depend on eating any source of nutrients we can get. While the word *sparingly* certainly encompasses "not abundantly," given verses 13 and 15, I wonder if in this context the word *sparingly* may mean *as little as is needed.*

If the Lord were to ask us to discipline our children *sparingly*, we would probably not assume that we had to discipline them at least a little, regardless of their behavior. We would not feel we had to punish them, at least a little, even if they were perfectly obedient. No, we would understand that we should discipline them *as little as is needed* and, when not needed, not at all.

We are instructed to eat meat sparingly, but we are further told that it is pleasing to the Lord that we not eat meat at all, except under certain conditions. While there have been several alternative explanations of verse 13 since the Word of Wisdom was revealed in 1833, so far none of them stand up to careful analysis.[2] Maybe we should consider taking the Lord at His word.

## Do We Need to Consume Animal Foods?

Why would the Word of Wisdom instruct us to avoid animal flesh as a featured part of our diet if, as we are taught, animal foods are an important part of a balanced diet? Where can we get the nutrients to be healthy and strong if we don't regularly consume meat? Aren't there certain nutrients we *must* get from animal foods in order for our bodies to function optimally? Aren't meat and dairy two of the important food groups?

As we all know, the human body must have fuel to provide the energy needed for survival. Three macronutrients can provide energy: lipids (fats), proteins, and carbohydrates. In addition, micronutrients such as vitamins, minerals, and phytochemicals are vital for a host of bodily functions on every level.

What I learned took me by surprise. I discovered that *plants* (not animals) are the original source of *all* of the essential macro- *and* micronutrients the human body needs. Food science expert Harold McGee explains:

> Unlike animals, plants can synthesize organic materials from the minerals, air, and sunlight, and so they are the true origin of the proteins, carbohydrates, and other complex molecules necessary to animal life.[3]

Plants are the original source of all the dietary nutrients needed by our bodies:

- All the essential amino acids needed to build **protein**.
- All the essential **fatty acids** (omega 3 and omega 6).
- All **carbohydrates** (the human body's preferred fuel source).
- All the required **vitamins** or building blocks needed to produce the vitamins (with the exception of vitamins B12 or D, neither of which—with very rare exception—is created by plants or animals).[4]
- All the essential **minerals** (which plants absorb from the soil).

In addition, plants provide a rich abundance of other nutrients that produce optimal human health. For example,

- **Phytochemicals**, including antioxidants (thousands of phytochemicals function in various ways to fight disease and maintain health in our bodies).
- **Fiber** (essential for bodily functions, eliminating toxins, and healthy weight).
- **Water** (next to oxygen, the most essential element to life; food high in water helps cleanse the body and maintain healthy weight).

Not only do plants provide the nutrients needed for optimal health, they naturally provide these nutrients in the proportions needed by our bodies. Given the total number of calories required to build and fuel our bodies, we need no more than 10 percent of our calories from proteins[5] and no more than 10 percent of our calories from fats,[6] and most of us require even less. If we consume no animal foods and mostly low-fat whole plant foods, almost any plant-based diet (aside from an all-fruit diet) would still consist of at least 10 percent protein and 10 percent fat. In others words, assuming we are getting an adequate number of calories, plants naturally contain all of the proteins and fats we require for optimal health, without our having to go to special lengths to make sure we are getting enough in the right combinations. No wonder plants are ordained of God for the "constitution" and "nature" of His children (D&C 89:10).

## A Backup Source of Nutrition

If plants provide all that is needed to not only sustain human life but also to optimize our health, what is the role of animal flesh in our diet? Like us, animals get their essential nutrients from plants. Even the carnivorous animals at the top of the food chain ultimately depend totally on plant foods, as plants are the beginning of the food chain. But like us, most animals can get all the nutrients they need for optimal health from a vegetarian diet. The largest land mammals on the planet (elephants, giraffes, rhinos, hippopotamuses, and water buffalo) are all herbivores; *they eat only plant foods*. Humans are omnivores; we can get our nutrients from both plants and animals, but animal foods are *completely optional* for human nutrition. The fact that plants alone can nourish the largest, strongest land animals should help us understand how an all-plant diet can grow and maintain our much smaller human bodies.

As animals eat plants, vital nutrients become part of their bodies. Therefore, in times of necessity, when we humans can't get enough plants to sustain life (for example, in times of famine or excess cold when plants are scarce), we can eat animals as a backup source of nutrition. They have enough of the essential nutrients in their bodies, along with the needed calories, to sustain our lives in times of need.

However, eating animal foods comes at a price since the nutrients in them are not packaged ideally for regular human consumption. For example, when we get our nutrients from animal foods (including fish[7]), we also get

- **Too much cholesterol** (the human body produces all the cholesterol we need to function optimally, so *any* animal cholesterol is in excess of our needs and large quantities can be detrimental to our health).
- **Too much protein** (extra animal protein forces our livers and kidneys to work harder to process the excess, increases the acid load in our bodies, and creates an environment more conducive to cancer growth).
- **Too much fat** (and usually the wrong types of fat—saturated fat instead of the healthier unsaturated fats, like omega 3).
- **Too few of most essential nutrients: vitamins and minerals.**

- **Too much of some nutrients** (like iron, which is more easily absorbed when packaged in animal foods, contributing to various chronic illnesses).
- **No phytochemicals** ("phyto" means *plants*; they help us maintain health).
- **No carbohydrates,** aside from lactose (100 percent of meat calories come from protein and fat).
- **No dietary fiber** (a lack of fiber in the diet promotes constipation and fatigue and diminishes healthy gut bacteria).
- **Too many hormones, antibiotics,** etc. (both natural hormones and drugs given to animals to make them grow fast and keep them from getting sick).
- **Too many pollutants, microbes, pesticides, herbicides,** etc. (these get concentrated in animal foods because they are higher-up on the food chain).

Plants contain all the advantages with none of these disadvantages. In short, animal foods are in no way more ideal for the human body than plant foods, but they are a good backup source of nutrition. Perhaps this is one reason the Lord ordained them for our "use" under certain conditions, but not for the "constitution" or "nature" of our bodies (D&C 89:10-13).

## Where Do You Get Your Protein?

Anyone who stops eating animal foods will soon discover that other people, even strangers, are suddenly concerned they are not consuming enough protein. People who know little about nutrition nevertheless know that our bodies require protein, that it must be "complete" (that is, contain all of the essential amino acids), and that animal flesh contains a high percent of complete protein. All of this is true. What most people do not know is that protein is so ubiquitous in plant foods that if you get a sufficient number of calories, it is almost impossible not to get enough protein, including all the essential amino acids.[8] You do not need to pay attention to the amount and type of amino acids in the foods you eat.

Protein is essential to life, but like oxygen, it is so readily available we don't need to worry about where we are going to get it. We can't live for more than a few minutes without oxygen, but unlike aquatic mammals, we don't store large quantities in our bodies because we are built for an environment with plenty of oxygen. Likewise, our bodies don't store an excess of protein because they are built for an environment with plenty of protein. In fact, in our society we are more in danger of consuming too *much* protein than too little.

Furthermore, I learned that the idea that animal protein is superior to plant protein is a myth. Research indicates the opposite is true. Plant proteins are better for both the normal functioning of the human body and for warding off disease. Studies of human populations demonstrate a strong correlation between animal protein and a host of chronic diseases. While correlation is not causation, controlled studies indicate that animal protein is a causal factor in chronic illness. For example, cancer cells grow faster in a high animal protein environment. As T. Colin Campbell documents in *The China Study*, one can control the growth of cancer in rats by adjusting the percentage of animal protein in their diet. Vegetable protein does not have the same effect.[9] Animals do not need to eat complete proteins for their health requirements; their bodies take the various amino acids from various plants to produce the precise combinations they need. Our human bodies do the same. We do not need animals to process our proteins any more than we need the food industry to process our carbs or our fats. Our bodies are built to process all the needed carbs, fats, and proteins from the original source of these nutrients: plants. Even when we eat animals, our bodies break down their amino acids and re-combine them for our use.

Since most Americans consume animal foods, it is no surprise that the typical American consumes far more protein (approximately 17 percent of calories) than is needed. Animal foods are also high in fat, and with the addition of highly processed plant foods, fat now constitutes an incredible 35 percent of calories in the average American diet. In the case of both fat and protein, consuming more than we need is not a bonus; in fact, it can be harmful to our health, not to mention our waistlines. Every modern society that has seen an increase in the amount of protein and fat in their diets has seen a concomitant rise in chronic illness of every kind.[10] More is not better. More is killing us.

## Should We Never Eat Animals?

Despite the problems with animal foods, they can be lifesaving in times of need, just as the Lord ordained. Think of Lehi and his family eating raw meat in the wilderness as they travelled to the promised land or a pioneer family killing a buffalo as they crossed the plains. Animal foods provide a *backup* source of nutrition in times of necessity, and in these times we should use them "with thanksgiving," as the Word of Wisdom admonishes.

I don't call myself a "vegan" because my focus is not just on avoiding animal foods; my focus is on eating the foods that are best for my body. I don't believe I'm condemned if I eat some animal foods, whether by mistake or as a rare choice. And, because of the Word of Wisdom, I'm glad to know God ordained animals to save my life in case of need. I'd be supremely grateful to eat meat to keep from starvation or even severe hunger, but in all my life this has never been the reason I have ever eaten even a single piece of meat. I have always had plenty and enough to spare, with modern heating and clothing to prevent me from truly experiencing winter or cold, and with enough grocery stores, refrigerators, and restaurants to make food far too plentiful for optimal health. I'm grateful now to refrain from eating meat when there is no need, knowing this is pleasing to the Lord. I believe the Word of Wisdom is also telling me this is best for my body. Surprisingly, it took science to help me see and appreciate these words of wisdom.

Regardless of exactly how we interpret the Word of Wisdom, D&C 89 clearly comes down strongly on the "low-protein" side of the nutritional debate. Plenty of high-protein proponents, both before and after Robert Atkins, have claimed that science is on their side. No amount of evidence contrary to their position seems to dissuade them. To the layperson, the scientific evidence may seem inconclusive, but I believe the Word of Wisdom helps us sort fact from fiction. The Atkins diet and other high-protein or low-carbohydrate diets may help some people lose weight (as almost any diet will), but they don't measure up to the standard set by the Word of Wisdom. Therefore, I give more credence to the substantial amount of scientific evidence (see Appendix Seven) that concludes such diets have a significantly negative effect on our health in the long run. I don't want to gamble on my health by betting against the Word of Wisdom.

## Keeping the Word of Wisdom

Let me state here for the record that I do not think Latter-day Saints must avoid eating all meat in order to "keep the Word of Wisdom." The Lord's servants have defined obedience to the Word of Wisdom as abstaining from alcohol, tobacco, coffee, tea, illegal drugs, and habit-forming substances.[11] This book is not about changing this definition. I whole-heartedly sustain this standard, which I believe has been set by divine inspiration. I am in no position to propose (nor do I desire to campaign) that the standard be changed. According to my understanding, all who abstain from these harmful substances are "keeping the Word of Wisdom" as far as what we have been asked to do.

What I do suggest is that the Lord gives us much more advice in Section 89 that can also bless our lives. The blessings promised in D&C 89 apply to all the counsel given in that section of scripture, not just to the prohibitions. In a sense, there are two meanings to the phrase *Word of Wisdom*. One is the standard the Church has set for worthiness to become a member of the LDS Church and remain worthy to participate in all the ordinances. The other refers to the totality of guidance given in D&C 89. Both meanings are commonly used among Latter-day Saints. Please keep in mind that in this book when I refer to the Word of Wisdom, I am using the *broader* meaning, but I do not confuse that broader meaning with the narrower, *more important*, standard set by Church leaders.

---

# Real Mormons ✨ Real Stories

## *Debbie's Story*

I am a registered dietitian. I have been passionate about nutrition for as long as I can remember, especially as it relates to the Word of Wisdom. As I raised my family, I read and re-read this revelation to find the best way to feed them. I always felt some concern about the admonition to eat meat "sparingly" and thought I was doing a pretty good job when I cut the meat in a recipe down from one pound to half a pound. Nonetheless, I admit I was biased in my thoughts and attitude about vegetarians and vegans, believing their diets to be too extreme. No one could be more surprised than me that I now eat a whole food, plant-based diet!

My journey into the world of plant-based eating started several years ago when I walked into a Sam's Club with my friend, Ilene Christensen, and discovered they were performing free cholesterol screenings. We decided to have ours checked. Ilene's cholesterol was 238 and mine was 201, which put us at risk for heart disease.

As a dietitian I was dismayed for both of us. I didn't know anyone who ate "healthier" than we did or who worked out harder than Ilene. She asked me if her cholesterol was bad, and I told her that if she had been at her doctor's office instead of at Sam's, she would have been given a prescription for Lipitor, especially considering that her father died of a heart attack when he was only 46. She asked what she could do to lower her cholesterol, and my answer was that she was already doing all of the things any dietitian would tell her to do. I told her to make an appointment with her doctor.

Ilene didn't like my answer and did some personal research. She bought a book about eating a whole food, plant-based diet written by an MD. My initial reaction to the book was skepticism because a doctor had written it. I told her I didn't read diet books written by doctors who had minimal to no nutrition background because they wrote really bad stuff like *Dr. Atkins' New Diet Revolution.*

Ilene finally convinced me to read the book, and it made sense—a lot of sense. As I compared it to the Word of Wisdom, I found no contradictions. In fact, it followed the Word of Wisdom precisely! We decided to give the advice in the book a six-week trial to see if we could actually eat plant-based and to see if it made a difference in our health. During that six-week period I also read *The China Study* by T. Colin Campbell—twice. The book literally changed my life! I was more determined than ever to live a whole food, plant-based lifestyle for the rest of my life. Incidentally, after our six weeks was up, we retested our cholesterol. Ilene went from a cholesterol reading of 238 to 164 and mine went from 201 to 138. Plus, we both lost about 15 pounds!

In *The China Study*, Dr. Campbell talks about making paradigm shifts. Most of us have to reconcile this new information with what we believed to be true for so many years. My own paradigm shift came in bits and pieces. For instance, a really big shift came very early in my WFPB adventure when Ilene asked me which had more protein, broccoli or steak. I looked at her as though she had lost her mind. Clearly she had to know that steak was the protein food! When she announced she had discovered that, calorie for calorie, broccoli had more protein than some cuts of steak, I was astounded. How could a dietitian NOT know that?! But I didn't know! I began to wonder what else I didn't know and started searching in earnest for answers to questions I had not known to ask.

Years ago I set a lifelong goal to go throughout life with healthy measures for weight, cholesterol, blood pressure, and glucose, all without medication. Yet no matter how hard I tried to eat "right" and how hard I worked out, I was still battling my weight. In addition, my blood pressure and cholesterol readings kept going up. I was beginning to believe my goal would be impossible to maintain. When my whole food, plant-based eating brought all of those numbers back into control, I experienced two initial and extreme emotions. First, I was elated and overjoyed that I had found something so simple that made such a big difference. Next, I became incredibly angry with my profession and our entire medical society. Why didn't I learn about plant-based eating as an option for health in my dietetics studies? Why did it seem that everyone in authority was keeping so many basic truths from the American public? For a time, I actually felt embarrassed to put the RD credentials behind my name because I believed they represented something of a lie.

As the years have gone by and my anger has subsided, I have found ways to make a difference in my profession. I am now an instructor for the T. Colin Campbell Foundation, which offers a Certificate in Plant-based Nutrition through eCornell. I am still passionate about nutrition. In fact, my passion is stronger now than ever, and I love sharing this message with anyone who will listen. I thank my Heavenly Father every day for my vibrant health, that I was led to discover the "hidden treasures" of a whole food, plant-based way of eating, and for the comfort of promised blessings found in the Word of Wisdom.

*Debbie Christofferson, age 59, lives in Hyde Park, Utah. She is a faculty member in the Nutrition, Dietetics, and Food Science Department at Utah State University and teaches the Plant-Based Nutrition course from eCornell. She has four children and ten grandchildren. She loves to cook, read, and travel.*

Debbie's friend, Ilene Christensen, has her story featured on the website discoveringthewordofwisdom.com.

# 3

# Wholesome Herbs and Every Fruit

Of course, the counsel about animal flesh is just one part of the Word of Wisdom. The other injunctions are equally interesting:

> And again, verily I say unto you, all wholesome herbs God hath ordained for the constitution, nature, and use of man— Every herb in the season thereof, and every fruit in the season thereof; all these to be used with prudence and thanksgiving. (D&C 89:10–11)

We typically think of herbs as plants with specific culinary or medicinal purposes, but the D&C footnote to these verses suggests the word *herbs* means simply *plants*. The 1828 *Webster's Dictionary* states, "The word herb comprehends all the grasses, and numerous plants used for culinary purposes." *Webster's* defines *fruit* generally as "whatever the earth produces for the nourishment of animals," including "all cultivated plants," and more narrowly as

> the produce of a tree or other plant; the last production for the propagation or multiplication of its kind; the seed of plants, or the part that contains the seeds; as wheat, rye, oats, apples, quinces, pears, cherries, acorns, melons, [etc.].

The phrasing of this Word of Wisdom injunction echoes the admonition given to Adam and Eve in the Garden of Eden:

> And God said, Behold, I have given you every herb bearing seed, which is upon the face of all the earth, and every tree, in

the which is the fruit of a tree yielding seed; to you it shall be for meat. (Genesis 1:29)

The Hebrew word for *herb* in this verse is ê·śeḇ, meaning plants. In fact, many Bible translators use the word *plants* in their translation of this verse:

Then God said, Behold, I have given you every plant yielding seed that is on the surface of all the earth, and every tree which has fruit yielding seed; it shall be food for you. (*New American Standard Bible*, 1995)

The Word of Wisdom specifies we are to eat all "wholesome" plants. The word *wholesome* means "tending to promote health; favoring health" (1828 *Webster's Dictionary*). In other words, all health-promoting plants are ordained "for the *constitution, nature, and use* of man" (emphasis added). As noted previously, this wording contrasts with verse 12 in which the flesh of beasts is ordained for "the *use* of man" without mention of it being ordained either for our *constitution* or *nature,* as are plants. Indeed, plants do form the very constitution or nature of our bodies as the molecules, cells, proteins, and enzymes that make up our bodies come from the plants of this earth. What a sacred role plants were given to become the very tabernacles of God's children! The power of the sun, the moon, and the stars, along with the vitality of earth, water, air, and fire all come together in our bodies via plants!

We know that not just Adam and Eve, but also every beast, fowl, and creeping thing were given plants to eat in the Garden of Eden, and because death had not yet come into the world, all living things were vegetarian, just as they will apparently be in the Millennium when

The wolf and the lamb shall feed together, and the lion shall eat straw like the bullock: and dust shall be the serpent's meat. They shall not hurt nor destroy in all my holy mountain, saith the Lord. (Isaiah 65:25)

I have no idea how this works in terms of the physiology of carnivorous animals, but it seems clear that the meat-eating ways of human beings will one day come to an end. I also believe that the Word of Wisdom suggests what science confirms: *plants are the optimal food for human beings.* History provides supporting evidence: as a youth, the prophet Daniel and his Hebrew friends in captivity refused the rich meaty food of the King and asked to be served pulse and water (that is, a vegetarian diet),[1] resulting in their visibly greater health (see Daniel 1).

Whole plants are the goldmines of nutrition. They transform the power of the sun, the soil, water, and air to produce the macro- and micronutrients required by the human body, indeed for all animal life. It's not just the vitamins, minerals, fatty acids, protein, water, and fiber—it is also a wide range of phytochemicals: alkaloids, carotenoids, flavonoids, isoflavones, organosulfides, phenolic acids, phytosterols, saponins, and many more that have and have not yet been discovered.[2] Plant foods are so packed with nutrients that promote health and guard against disease that scientists have barely begun to uncover the power they contain and the beautifully complex and symbiotic ways they work together at every level in our bodies. But while we do not know everything, we do know a diet rich in plants helps prevent most of the chronic illnesses that plague us.[3]

## What about Processed Plant Foods?

While the Word of Wisdom does not explicitly state that plants should only be eaten in their whole, unrefined forms, the word *wholesome* arguably points in this direction, and common sense confirms this is optimal. If God packaged plant foods with such a large number and variety of powerful nutrients and phytochemicals that modern scientists are only beginning to understand what they are and how they work together to keep our bodies strong and healthy, why would it make sense to consume foods that are largely stripped of these nutrients? Likewise, why would it be better to isolate and concentrate nutrients into supplements in place of consuming them in the infinitely more complex, balanced combinations that naturally occur in whole foods? Science confirms that the original state of plants and nutrients is best for our bodies.[4] While explicit reference to processed foods is absent from the Word of Wisdom, we are admonished to eat "wholesome" plants "with prudence" (v. 11). I'm not sure turning strawberries into Strawberry Splash Fruit Gushers quite meets that standard.

Confining our diet to "plant foods" is not enough for good health. After all, many junk foods are wholly, or nearly wholly, derived from plants. Even if they are "vegetarian," we all know human bodies are not made to thrive on Pringles, Ritz Crackers, or Pop-Tarts. When plants are heavily processed, so many nutrients are taken out that the end so-called "food" product is often mere empty calories (supplying energy to the body without any of the needed micronutrients). Worse, because these refined foods are so different in composition from what our bodies thrive on, they can actually do us harm. Think about the difference between beets and beet sugar, between corn and corn oil, between asparagus (with 33 percent of its calories from protein) and asparagus protein powder (I'm making this one up, but you get the idea!).

We are admonished to eat "wholesome" plants with "prudence." The 1828 *Webster's* definition of prudence is "Wisdom applied to practice." Further, *Webster's* explains:

> Prudence implies caution in deliberating and consulting on the most suitable means to accomplish valuable purposes, and the exercise of sagacity in discerning and selecting them. Prudence differs from wisdom in this, that prudence implies more caution and reserve than wisdom, or is exercised more in foreseeing and avoiding evil, than in devising and executing that which is good.

To use wholesome plants with "prudence" implies exercising great judgment and wisdom in carefully deciding how to use that which the Lord has provided for our health. If any adjective more soundly contradicts the way most of us Americans choose to eat, I can't think of one. I wonder how it can ever be "prudent" to strip plant foods of their vital nutrients so we can indulge our love for yummy-tasting junk food at the expense of our health? And yet I have to confess this was largely my pattern of eating for most of my life.

Another clue to the wisdom of not using heavily processed foods is found in the phrase that admonishes us to eat plants "in the season thereof." An important purpose for processing and refining food is so that the food will have a long shelf life for cost-efficiency and so we can eat them out of season. But as Michael Pollan points out, "Real food is alive—and therefore it should eventually die."[5] Processing can add months, even years to the shelf life of foods, but it does so at the expense of many of their shelf-unstable nutrients. Processing also allows the addition of food additives, fats, salts, and sugars that can be harmful to our bodies, as well as preservatives that allow us to eat them well past "the season thereof."

Some processing of food is inevitable and doesn't do much harm; chopping up vegetables is a form of processing them. Some processing can even be beneficial (e.g., some vitamins are more accessible when food is cooked). Certainly canning, freezing, and preserving whole ripe plants "in the season thereof" is an excellent option and prudent for helping us prepare for times of need. But extensive processing is problematic.[6]

Aside from a loss of some nutrients, why would a food be any less good for our bodies just because it is highly processed? One reason is that the more a food is processed, the more the sugar, salt, and fat are concentrated in the food, and the more these ingredients are concentrated, the more addictive the food becomes. This explains why the exact same molecules (e.g., glucose and fructose) that are not addictive in whole foods (like beets and corn) are addictive in the form of table sugar and Jolly Ranchers. Registered dietitian Jeff Novick explains:

> The answer has to do with concentration. Same as with cocaine. Coca leaves are not very addictive. Cocaine, a more concentrated form, has a much higher potential for addiction. Crack, a much more concentrated form, is much more highly addictive.[7]

Is there any doubt that junk foods are addictive in a way spinach and strawberries are not? I don't feel I'm going out on a limb when I suggest that potato chips don't qualify under "wholesome" plants. And this undoubtedly applies to many other modern foods, even if they are not spelled out in Section 89. When asked why the Lord does not give us further guidance on the many different drinks and foods not specifically addressed in the Word of Wisdom, President Joseph Fielding Smith stated:

> Such revelation is unnecessary . . . If we sincerely follow what is written with the aid of the Spirit of the Lord, we need no further counsel . . . we are promised inspiration and the guidance of the Spirit of the Lord through which we will know what is good and what is bad for the body, without the Lord presenting us with a detailed list separating the good things from the bad. . . .
>
> A safe guide to each and all is this: If in doubt as to any food or drink, whether it is good or harmful, let it alone until you have learned the truth in regard to it.[8]

Elder Boyd K. Packer warned:

> There are many habit-forming, addictive things that one can drink or chew or inhale or inject which injure both body and spirit which are not mentioned in the [Word of Wisdom].[9]

Yes, it is true, for example, that the Word of Wisdom "does not mention the use of caffeine."[10] It doesn't need to. If we have learned from personal experience or research that a substance is not good for us, it doesn't need to be spelled out for us. If we are concerned only about obeying the narrow definition of the Word of Wisdom, we know the bishop will not ask us whether we consume caffeine, doughnuts, meat, or other junk foods, but if we want better health, we had better seek the "inspiration and the guidance of the Spirit of the Lord" as we study the Word of Wisdom.

# What about Refined Plant Oils?

The advantages of eating whole, unrefined plant foods suggest that even so-called "heart-healthy" olive oil is not the best choice, even if it is extra virgin. Vegetable oils are among the most heavily processed, refined foods we routinely eat. At 4,000 calories per pound, they are also among the most calorically dense foods on earth. They provide close to zero nutritional benefit of any kind. Like sugar, they are "empty calories," but each gram is more than twice as fattening as sugar. In days gone by, fats were prized because calories were scarce, but in a world where most of us don't need any extra calories, this is no longer an advantage.

Just as processing whole plants into white flour and white sugar turns healthy foods into unhealthy ones, processing whole plants into oils does the same thing. This includes refined oils such as corn, soybean, olive, canola, and coconut oil. Whole sweet corn is roughly 80 percent carbohydrates, 10 percent fat and 10 percent protein. One cup of sweet corn is about 130 calories and contains all kinds of vitamins and minerals. Two tablespoons of corn oil, on the other hand, are almost 250 calories of 100 percent fat with very close to zero nutrients of any kind.

Whole green olives are almost 90 percent fat, but at least they contain a variety of nutrients and some fiber; 100 grams of pickled olives (3.5 ounces) clock in at 150 calories. If we squeeze out the fat from many olives to produce just 28 grams of olive oil (two tablespoons), we discard almost all of the nutrients and all of the fiber, and we are left with 100 percent pure fat that clocks in at about 240 calories, including 14 percent saturated fat. At 90 percent saturated fat, coconut oil is even worse, notwithstanding its current popularity as a "health" food.[11]

Vegetable oils are not whole foods; they are pure fat, and fat is simply not a nutrient we need more of. There are only two essential fats, namely the fatty acids called omega 3 and omega 6, which our bodies cannot make. The amount of these fats our bodies need is very, very small, and we get all we need from eating a natural variety of whole-plant foods. Adding vegetable oil only adds unneeded calories.[12]

What about all the studies that link the use of olive oil, coconut oil, or other oils with better heath? Refined oils only appear healthy in contrast to fats that are even worse for our bodies. If we use vegetable oils *in place of* more damaging fats, we may see benefits, but to add them to a whole food, plant-based diet makes the diet worse, not better, for our health. There is no benefit to adding refined fat to a healthy diet, and there are negative consequences. I'll share just two examples I find interesting. Modern technology can detect, in real time, the damage olive oil does to the endothelial lining of our arteries by measuring the arterial blood flow in people who have just consumed it. Monkeys fed monounsaturated fat (like olive oil) do show lower levels of bad cholesterol and higher levels of good cholesterol, but autopsies show that they develop just as much coronary artery disease as those who consume saturated fat.[13]

Refined oils are the junk calories of the fats, just as refined sugars are the junk calories of the carbohydrates. I found it surprisingly easy to do without vegetable oils when I switched to my new diet. Even with the serious lack of cooking skills I possessed, it was not difficult to learn to cook without them. That doesn't mean I believe we have to abstain from all oils in the same way we abstain from all alcohol or tobacco! I don't think we need to assiduously avoid every drop of vegetable oil, any more than we need to avoid all white flour or all white sugar. But if we use any of these refined foods, it should be because we think they are useful for flavor or convenience and *not* because they are "healthy." Nevertheless, how much better to eat *wholesome plants* in their *season* "with prudence and thanksgiving" (D&C 89:10–11).

## Real Mormons ❧ Real Stories

### *Ginger's Story*

At 35, I was a vegetarian with a very low iron count. My doctor said I needed to start eating meat, because my levels were dangerously low. Even though I knew it didn't follow the Word of Wisdom, I began cooking in a style similar to *Nourishing Traditions* and Fanny Farmer—with lots of white flour, sugar, butter, cream, cheese, and meat. I even wrote a great cookbook along those lines. Everyone loved my cooking—some of my children wax sentimental to this day when they talk about those years. My iron count remained low, but my cholesterol levels and weight soared; my moods were on a roller coaster.

Then at age 43, I got really ill. It started with what I thought was the flu, but it never went away—it was hypoadrenalism. This "flu" exacerbated my chronic constipation, chronic UTI, arthritis, acne, Raynaud's syndrome, intestinal bleeding, angina, anemia, PMS, eczema, blood sugar issues, emotional issues, and so on and so forth. I prayed and prayed to Heavenly Father to end my suffering and allow me to die in my sleep. He did end my suffering but not through death.

Because I've had some pretty bad experiences with medical doctors, I felt inspired to study herbalism instead. Through my classes, which I did from my bed, I was introduced to Dr. Christopher's *Mucusless Diet*, Boutenko's *Green For Life*, Dr. Fuhrman's *Eat to Live*, and Dr. Campbell's *The China Study*. After I finally put my resistance to veganism aside, I dove in headfirst. Since I had been an ovo-lacto vegetarian [eating eggs and dairy but no meat] nearly 100 percent of the time since age 16 (meat is so gross), eating lots of fruit, grains, and beans was easy. However, I never did learn to like many vegetables. I pretended to love all of them in front of my children, while swallowing them whole to avoid the taste.

Within a few weeks of beginning the *Eat to Live* diet, the constipation, UTI, acne, eczema, PMS, emotional issues, Raynaud's, and blood sugar imbalances were gone. However, fatigue, anemia, intestinal bloating/bleeding, angina, and arthritis played hide-and-seek over and over. Just when I thought I was all better, I'd be slammed back into bed. Because I was inspired along this path, I knew a low-fat, whole food, plant-based diet was right for me. However, even though I followed the Word of Wisdom, I didn't have the miraculous recovery others claimed. Not only could I not walk without fainting, I certainly could not run. Sometimes I couldn't even get out of bed. It was very discouraging.

I studied the Word of Wisdom closer and clung to verse 13, "And it is pleasing unto me that they [flesh foods] should NOT be used, ONLY in times of winter, or of cold, or famine," (D&C 89:13, emphasis added). Also, I began searching the Internet for anything on the subject of low-fat, plant-based nutritional healing and learned Dr. Fuhrman wasn't the only game in town. Although I'll forever be grateful to him, I learned new things from Dr. McDougall, Dr. Esselstyn, Jeff Novick, and the others in this camp. Finally, I read in "Diet: Only Hope for Arthritis" on Dr. McDougall's site about the link between increased intestinal permeability, food allergies, and arthritis. At last, I stepped toward healing. After a 12-week juice fast, I put pain and fatigue behind me. The fast allowed my intestines to heal, my inflammation to reverse, my adrenals to rest, and my body to absorb nutrients it desperately needed.

Oh, but I got thin, sooo thin. Adding in more grains and beans according to Dr. McDougall, while maintaining my use of pounds and pounds of veggies and fruit daily, has been the answer. My adrenals will never be 100 percent, but I don't have nearly as much trouble with symptoms of hypoadrenalism. With more energy, color in my cheeks, and no pain, I am a healthy weight and very happy almost 50-year-old grandma . . . if I don't allow temptation to convince me to eat one of my allergens: dairy, eggs, animal flesh and fats, wheat, soy, all oils, olives, some nuts, and some seeds.

A couple weeks ago I thought to myself, I must be some sort of hypochondriac and can't possibly be allergic to all those things. I ate what I shouldn't have. After a few days of this behavior, I couldn't walk and slept for days. Angina and inflammation came roaring back as well. Now, I'm a lifetime convert and eat to live according to the Word of Wisdom. Not only does it please the Savior that I don't use animal flesh except in a famine, I'm so much healthier and happier because of this inspired choice. I'll ever be grateful for this answer to my prayers. I absolutely love vegetables now!

*Ginger Conrad is 49 and lives in the Northwest United States. She and her husband enjoy their many children and grandchildren. She is a certified Montessori teacher and herbalist. For personal fulfillment, she likes to hike in the forest with her husband, do yoga, garden indoors, play the violin, and teach Primary.*

# 4

# All Grain Is Good

The following is one of my favorite injunctions in the Word of Wisdom:

> All *grain* is ordained for the use of man and of beasts, to be
> *the staff of life*. (D&C 89:14, emphasis added)

The "staff of life" means *staple of diet*. What is a staple? According to *Merriam-Webster*, the word *staple* used as a noun means "the sustaining or principal element" and "something having widespread and constant use or appeal." When used as an adjective, it means "principal, chief" and "used, needed, or enjoyed constantly usually by many individuals."[1] According to the Word of Wisdom, the principal element of our diet should be grains. Grains include grasses like wheat and rice, but corn and legumes (like beans, lentils, peas, and other pulses) can also be classified as grains.

I've been looking at this verse with a new perspective ever since I learned that the whole food, plant-based diet I discovered is also called a "starch-based diet" because the bulk of the calories come from starches. Since grains are the primary source of nutritional starch, a whole food, plant-based diet is a *grain-based diet*. This matches the wisdom of D&C 89:14 beautifully. Unsurprisingly, the idea of a grain-based diet is not new with the Word of Wisdom. John A. McDougall, MD, notes that, "Throughout civilization and around the world, six foods have provided our primary fuel: barley, maize (corn), millet, potatoes, rice, and wheat."[2] Dr. McDougall explains:

> All large populations of trim, healthy people, throughout
> verifiable human history, have obtained the bulk of their cal-
> ories from starch. Examples of once thriving people include

Japanese, Chinese, and other Asians eating sweet potatoes, buckwheat, and/or rice; Incas in South America eating potatoes; Mayans and Aztecs in Central America eating corn; and Egyptians in the Middle East eating wheat.[3]

I love that the wisdom of Section 89 has withstood the test of time and is nothing like a fad diet.

Why are grains so important? Why does it matter where we get our calories as long as they are whole foods? Allow me to explore one possible reason. As I mentioned, the world's largest land mammals are strictly vegetarian, but in order to consume enough calories, many of them must spend much of their day eating. If we did that, we would have little time for education, the arts, or even religious practice. The cultivation of grains through agriculture, therefore, is the foundation of civilization in the history of the human race. Grains and other starchy plant foods provide significantly more calories than the typical vegetable or even fruit, allowing humans to satisfy their energy requirements in a much more efficient way. These foods can also be more easily stored away for use in times of cold or famine. Human civilization is not possible without the cultivation of grains. They are, indeed, the "staff of life." Food expert Harold McGee writes:

> It would be hard to overestimate the importance of grains and legumes in the life of our species ... [They] have played a crucial role in human nutrition and cultural evolution.... The culture of the fields made possible the culture of the mind.[4]

What was true in the distant past is also true of the recent past. McGee observed the following in the early 1980's:

> [Grains] provide the bulk of the caloric intake for much of the world's population: around 70% for Egypt and India, and near 80% in China, or between 2 and 3 times the average for the developed West. The cereals and legumes put together account for more than two thirds of the world's dietary protein. Even the industrial countries are fed indirectly by the huge amounts of corn, wheat, and soybeans on which their cattle, hogs, and chickens are raised. When we learn that the cereals are members of the grass family, we find new significance in the Old Testament prophet Isaiah's admonition, "All flesh is grass."[5]

If you pay much attention to nutrition, you know many so-called experts are anti-carbohydrate and, often vehemently, anti-grain.[6] Some go so far as to state that the human body has no need for carbohydrates. Wheat is almost always at the top of their hit list, notwithstanding the Lord declared "wheat for man" (D&C 89:17). When I hear experts rail against grain and wheat, I think of what Isaiah said, "Surely your turning of things upside down shall be esteemed as the potter's clay" (Isaiah 29:16).

It is common among low-carb and Paleo experts to declare the agricultural revolution a mistake, to insist that humans were never designed to eat grains and cereals, and that we can't achieve optimal health while eating these foods. This contradicts history, science, and common sense. Despite claims to the contrary, even Paleolithic peoples got the majority of calories from carbohydrates.[7] And the ancestors of Paleolithic peoples were nearly complete vegetarians.[8] We humans are agriculturalists, tilling the soil since the days of Adam and Eve (see Genesis 3:23). In the past, only small populations in non-typical outlying areas of the world have thrived on a diet more heavy in animal foods; for them it was a necessity. Human bodies are able to adapt to a diet heavy in animal foods, but that has never been optimal, and no large population has ever done it without the introduction of widespread chronic illness.

## When the Staff of Life Gets Displaced

Only privileged people in the past, and we comparatively wealthy moderns today, have had the option to get the bulk of our calories from sources besides grains and other starches. Carbohydrates are not just the preferred fuel sources for our bodies; they are also the preferred fuel sources for our pocketbooks and waistlines. In past civilizations, only the rich could get a disproportionate number of calories from either fat or protein, so only the rich got the associated chronic illnesses. Today, developed societies have grown wealthy enough to eat like the kings and queens of old, and so now the common man is also suffering and dying like the royalty of days gone by.

China is an example of a country that, until very recently, was largely protected from most Western chronic illnesses due to their rice-based diet. Many studies document their dramatically lower levels of chronic illness of all kinds.[9] But over the past few decades, the average wealth of the Chinese has risen dramatically, allowing them to consume more meat, dairy, fat, and sugar, which have replaced starch and fiber. A large-scale study reported in *The Journal of the American Medical Association* notes that while less than one percent of the Chinese population were diabetic in 1980, that number rose to 5.5 percent in 2000, 9.7 percent in 2007 and

11.6 percent in 2010.[10] At 11.6, the percentage of diabetics in China is now one of the highest in the world, surpassing even the United States. Clearly it isn't just the food, since their diet is still not as bad as ours. Some suggest that because their ancestors had to survive for long periods on very low food resources, peoples like the Chinese have developed "thrifty" genes, which allowed them to survive famines, but also made them particularly sensitive to chronic disease once introduced to a rich food environment. Sadly, we are also seeing this same skyrocketing rate of diabetes in other peoples with "thrifty" genes, like the Pima Indians in Arizona, as soon as they move away from their traditional grain-based diets.[11]

Humans are designed to thrive on a *starch-based* (complex carbohydrate) diet, not a protein-based diet or fat-based diet. We are not primarily meat, dairy, egg, or even nut or seed eaters. We are not even designed to thrive on a primarily vegetable- or fruit-based diet, raw or cooked, with or without green smoothies. Although most of us should consume a lot more raw fruits and vegetables, many people who "fail" on a vegetarian diet do so because they neglect to consume enough grains and then load up on other types of food that are not designed to be the staff of life.

While I do not doubt that certain individuals are sensitive to specific grains, and some are gluten intolerant or function best without wheat, the wholesale condemnation of grains goes against both human physiology and human history. The anti-grain rhetoric of low-carb, Paleo, and other anti-grain diets does not square with the Word of Wisdom. While non-Latter-day Saints have an excuse for being confused, we do not. We have been told by the best of sources, "All grain is ordained for the use of man . . . to be the staff of life" and "All grain is good for the food of man" (D&C 89:14 & 16).

## Wisdom Needed Especially in Our Day

I found it enlightening to learn that in societies where people consume a largely whole food, plant-based diet founded on grains as the staff of life, they suffer from relatively few of the chronic illnesses that plague our society today and that this was true of peoples of all the great civilizations of the past.[12] However, that does not mean they all enjoyed perfect health. In fact, on average, we enjoy better health than our ancestors did, even if our diet, in many respects, is worse. To understand why, we need to distinguish between two distinct types of diseases: *communicable* (infectious) and *noncommunicable*.

I am very grateful we do not live as our ancestors did, under the constant threat of ravaging diseases that swept through communities, killing and maiming huge numbers of people. These were primarily communicable diseases like the bubonic plague, diarrheal diseases, diphtheria, dysentery, influenza, malaria, smallpox, syphilis, tuberculosis, typhoid fever, and yellow fever. Other major killers in the past included hunger, childbirth, war, and accidents. Fortunately, we now know how to avert most of these tragedies, but our ancestors were relatively defenseless against many terrifying threats because they were often poor in sanitation, food security, and medical knowledge.

Even as late as the nineteenth century, when the Word of Wisdom was revealed, the greatest threats to human health were the infectious diseases, *not* the diet-related noncommunicable diseases which the Word of Wisdom seems tailor-made to address. If the Word of Wisdom had been primarily for the benefit of nineteenth-century Saints, it should have focused on issues of *sanitation*, not diet, in order to dramatically improve health conditions.[13] Even if the early Saints had followed the diet guidelines in Section 89 strictly (which they didn't), it would have had a relatively small impact on their health as compared to ours.

Because they were vulnerable to infectious diseases, many people before the twentieth century did not live long enough to reach the age where we tend to suffer from the noncommunicable chronic illnesses prevalent today, but *those who did live long enough were largely spared from these diseases.* These are the diseases that are diet and lifestyle-related. They include the host of common inflammatory diseases like heart disease, strokes, impotence, and kidney disease. They also include the various autoimmune diseases such as Crohn's disease, lupus, multiple sclerosis, arthritis, psoriasis, and thyroiditis. Furthermore, diabetes, asthma, hypertension, and obesity were virtually unknown in whole food, starch-based populations, and the incidence of various cancers was likewise low.

The Word of Wisdom dietary counsel is needed much more in our day than it was when it was first revealed. Only since the twentieth century have we had the wealth and resources to eradicate or control many of the terrifying infectious diseases of the past. But that same wealth has also allowed us to displace grain as the staff of life and put animal and other rich foods in its place. So just as our wealth has led to the eradication of infectious diseases and dramatically lengthened our lifespans, that wealth has led to more years spent suffering from the consequences of an increasingly rich diet.

While we have learned how to prevent and control communicable diseases, our society remains largely ignorant of the fact that the noncommunicable diseases are also preventable, and so we are still living in the dark. I believe the way we eat today and feed our children is the modern equivalent of our ancestors choosing to work with (and allowing their children to play with) people in the community with bubonic plague or typhoid fever. It took a herculean effort to come as far as we have in eradicating communicable diseases. Where is the societal resolve to stamp out the noncommunicable diseases?

Contrast the relative absence of noncommunicable diseases in starch-based societies with the United States, where more than 90 million Americans live with chronic illnesses, accounting for 70 percent of deaths and 75 percent of the medical care costs. According to the Centers for Disease Control and Prevention (CDC):

> Chronic diseases—such as cardiovascular disease (primarily heart disease and stroke), cancer, and diabetes—are among the most prevalent, costly, and preventable of all health problems. Seven of every ten Americans who die each year, or more than 1.7 million people, die of a chronic disease.[14]

While it is true that genes play a role in disease, they are not the primary cause. WFPB experts point out: *genes load the gun, but diet pulls the trigger.* We see this most clearly in numerous examples of people moving from one area of the world, where they consume a largely whole food, plant-based diet, to a developed country like America where they (and especially their children and grandchildren) consume more Western foods. With the change of diet comes a dramatic increase in the incidence of chronic illness.[15] *Their genes did not change; their diet did.*

For some time now, people in developed countries have been much more likely to die because of too *much* food rather than too *little* food. Sadly, this is also true of underdeveloped countries now that our disease-inducing diet is being adopted in parts of the world that previously ate a more healthy grain-based diet. In China, more than 80 percent of annual deaths are now due to noncommunicable chronic illnesses. What is worse, if they are not able to reverse the tide, "the prevalence of cardiovascular disease, chronic obstructive pulmonary disease, diabetes, and lung cancer in individuals older than 40 years will double or even triple during the next two decades."[16] Noncommunicable diseases are now the leading cause of death in every region of the world, except Africa (where they are projected to exceed other causes of death by 2030).[17]

We associate people who rely on grains as the staff of life with people who are relatively poor, those who can't afford rich processed and animal foods. Most poor people do not eat a diet of primarily grains and other plant foods for health reasons, but because that is all they can afford to eat or that is all they have access to. There have never been large populations who freely chose to be 100 percent vegetarian, much less vegan. Human beings enjoy eating meat and processed foods, and they almost invariably move toward making these foods the center of their meals when they are able. When we eat more of the calorically dense meat and processed foods, we inevitably eat less of something else, and that something else is usually the more calorically dense plant foods like whole grains. So as people gravitate toward animal and processed foods, these foods become, for them, the staff of life, displacing grains and other starches. Sadly, at the same time people are growing rich in the things of the world, the foods of affluence are making them poor in health. Much of their increased income may now have to be spent on medical bills.

I'm grateful for the Word of Wisdom, which contains the counsel and guidance we need in today's world to know what to consume and what not to consume so we can enjoy optimal health. In the past, our ancestors ate a diet largely of necessity, not of choice. In no other time in the history of humankind have we been able to so freely choose between so many harmful and healthful foods, *therefore, in no other time have we been in such great need of these words of wisdom.*

## Wisdom Needed for Our Future Survival

While we know the Word of Wisdom is important in addressing the noncommunicable diseases today, it may be equally as needed to combat communicable diseases in the future. While there are many sources for infectious disease, historically, animals have been the primary source. Pathogenic biological agents (disease-causing bugs) have been transmitted to humans through our close and constant contact with the animals we raised, or in our efforts to hunt wild animals for food.[18] The medical community has laudably developed powerful antibiotics to combat these diseases; however the intense, relentless use of antibiotics and other drugs, particularly in efforts to stimulate growth and ward off disease in animals raised for food around the world, are having the side effect of creating superbugs, which are antibiotic-resistant. These superbugs may one day be more powerful than every pharmaceutical drug we throw at them.[19] In a recent study conducted by Consumer Reports on ground turkey, "90% of the samples had one or more of the five bacteria for which [they] tested" and "almost all of the disease-causing organisms . . . proved resistant to one or more of the antibiotics commonly used to fight them." Consumer Reports linked the "speeding growth of drug-resistant superbugs" directly to the overuse of antibiotics in animals.[20] While part of the problem is misuse in humans, 70 percent of the antibiotics used in America are used for animals.[21]

Due to the overuse of antibiotics, some of the dreaded nineteenth-century diseases are coming back in versions that are resistant to drugs. Tuberculosis kills more people than any other treatable infectious disease, but now, in some parts of the world, 25 percent of the cases of tuberculosis are the multidrug-resistant form.[22] Over 23,000 Americans die each year from antibiotic-resistant infections.[23] More Americans succumb to antibiotic-resistant diseases than to HIV/AIDS.[24] At the same time this crisis is escalating, drug manufacturers are spending the bulk of their research dollars searching for drugs that treat noncommunicable diseases because the affluent can afford to make this research profitable. We don't have to rely on drugs for illnesses that are largely preventable through diet and lifestyle, but some of the infectious diseases are lethal (even to affluent Americans) without drugs that work.

One of the great blessings of the Word of Wisdom is the precious promise of protection it includes. If we only consumed animals in times of need, we would not have to raise them in a way that encourages the development of drug-resistant superbugs. If we ate a Word of Wisdom diet, we could dramatically increase our health and decrease human dependence on antibiotics, thus preserving their effectiveness for times when they are truly needed.

The Word of Wisdom was specifically designed for the "temporal salvation of all saints in the last days" (D&C 89:2). But Latter-day Saints are not the only ones who will benefit from this counsel. President Spencer W. Kimball stated, "We believe that the Lord, when he gave the Word of Wisdom, was speaking to all the people in the world."[25] Since there has never been a time in history when all the people in the world were in more need of these words of wisdom, let's make full use of the Lord's counsel and share it with others. Let's return to grains as the staff of life.

## Real Mormons ∽ Real Stories

### *Abbie's Story*

I met Jane Birch when my family moved to the US from South Korea twelve years ago. As their Young Women teacher, Jane kindly gave rides to my daughters to all YW activities and routinely visited my home to help them with their English, as well as their homework. Whenever she visited us, I fed her the Korean foods we usually ate. Gradually, I noticed her food preferences. She was not much in favor of our typical Korean foods, cooked with vegetables, seaweed, miso paste, and tofu. She liked meat marinated with sweet sauce (beef or pork bulgogi) and the sweet noodles (japchae) with beef. She sometimes tried a bite of some of our special Korean vegetables and then never touched them again. She called them "weeds."

My family did not eat much meat or sweets in Korea. Meat was expensive, so we enjoyed a lot of Korean dishes cooked with all kinds of vegetables, herbs, seaweed, beans, and tofu. And, like all Koreans, we ate lots and lots of rice: breakfast, lunch, and dinner. We enjoyed fruit as a dessert. Once in a while, on some special occasion, like one of my children's birthdays, I took them to a fancy Western restaurant in town and fed them pizza or spaghetti, thickly covered with Mozzarella cheese. A McDonald's hamburger was their favorite treat. In those days, I thought being westernized was a good thing. As a parent, I was so proud of myself that I could afford to treat my children to authentic Western food!! Even though I am LDS, I did not think about how much meat I ate in terms of the Word of Wisdom. Sometimes I did eat meat dishes, but they were a small portion of my diet. My family was healthy, and my children were beautiful and stayed in shape.

After we moved to the US, I was exposed to truly authentic American food. Instead of eating rice and tofu soup in the morning, we started to eat more eggs, bacon, sausage, and hash browns for breakfast. In place of our typical meal of rice, some kind of soup, and vegetable side dishes, we'd sometimes have pizza, hamburgers, pasta with Alfredo sauce (my favorite!), and lasagna, full of cheese. I started to cook a lot of meat dishes for my family and guests. I used plenty of butter and sugar. As Jane and I became friends, we hung out more often. She introduced me to all kinds of foods at all-you-can-eat buffets, Brazilian smorgasbords, westernized ethnic restaurants, and, of course, many ice cream parlors! I also discovered many new treats at almost every ward activity, like chocolate chip cookies and fudge-covered ice cream.

My tastes began to change. Even after eating Korean food, I felt like I needed a sweet dessert. Gradually I gained more than ten pounds. Worse, I felt tired all the time. My hands were stiff and swollen in the morning. I tried to exercise more, but my weight remained the same, and I did not feel healthy. I also started to worry about my children's eating habits, as they were eating more like Americans.

I was with Jane the morning she first learned about the "heart-attack proof" whole food, plant-based diet on CNN. Even though I was not happy with how I felt, I did not want to change my diet. I did not realize the importance of the food we eat every day. Also, I knew there are MANY man-made diet methods, and I did not want to chase them. When Jane was so determined to eat only plant-based food, I told her I would rather follow the Word of Wisdom, a diet God made, instead. I started to sincerely ponder each verse of D&C 89. I started to recognize what kind of food God wants to us eat. The sentence, "And it is pleasing unto me that they should not be used, only in times of winter, or of cold, or famine" struck me.

I started to cut down animal-based food: milk, cheese, meat, and egg. More than that, I cut down sweets (ice cream, cookies, cakes, and juices) and processed food, and I started to watch how much oil I was using. I began cooking more of the Korean foods I used to enjoy, with all kinds of vegetables, herbs, and beans. Now when Jane came to my house for dinner, she seemed to enjoy the traditional Korean foods much more. She even made me to teach her how to cook them!

Since I have returned to my traditional Korean diet, I have lost the weight I gained in America. My stiff hands are gone. I feel good when I eat more vegetable dishes, brown rice, and fruits. God promised that obedience to the Word of Wisdom would bring temporal and spiritual blessings. He also promised that the destroying angel (I think of this as chronic diseases like diabetes, heart disease, obesity, etc.) will pass us by and not slay us.

Fortunately, it was not too difficult for my husband and me to return to our Korean diet. It is not so easy for our four children. They love Korean food, but they are surrounded by cheap, convenient, highly caloric American foods of all kinds. It is a great temptation and an uphill battle. Yes, they "keep the Word of Wisdom," but I am praying that they will discover more of its meaning.

*Abbie (Gyungsook) Kim is 54 years old. After moving from South Korea to Utah in 2001, she studied nursing and earned an RN. She and her husband have four children, ages 31 to 23, and (almost) four grandchildren. They now live in the Chicago area, where they are blessed with even greater access to traditional Korean foods!*

# 5

# What about
# Dairy and Eggs?

D airy and eggs are not specifically mentioned in the Word of Wisdom—neither are Twinkies or Junior Mints. I conclude that none of these are as important to our health as are plants. Here, however, is an area where I realize I am stepping outside the wording of the Word of Wisdom to form an opinion. While WFPB experts feel the evidence is especially strong that dairy is one of the most unhealthy foods on the planet, the Word of Wisdom does not provide us with the same clear warning. Instead, as is so often the case with scripture, we must use our best judgment when it comes to discerning many of the practical implications of this revelation. In this case, I believe science provides us with ample evidence to help us study this question out in our minds. The following is my approach to the question of dairy and eggs.

While it is true that the Word of Wisdom does not specifically warn against dairy or eggs, it also includes absolutely nothing to promote their consumption. Instead, the Word of Wisdom counsels us to rely on plants (vegetables, fruits, and grains), and avoid the flesh of animals (except in times of need), for optimal health and spiritual blessings. Given the emphasis on the importance of plant foods and the admonition to use the flesh of animals only in times of need, on what basis would we conclude that consuming dairy or eggs would be wise for our health?

While there are some distinct differences, the nutritional profile of dairy and eggs is so similar to meat (and so distinct from plant foods) that we can consider them "liquid meat."[1] Like meat, dairy and eggs are not the original source of any essential nutrients. Like meat, dairy and eggs can provide nutrients to the human body, but they are not superior to plants in providing these nutrients, especially in light of the drawbacks. Like meat, the nutrients they do contain are packaged with much more that harms than helps our bodies (assuming we are not consuming them for survival reasons). Like meat, dairy and eggs contain too much protein, fat (especially saturated fat), cholesterol, calories, hormones, bacteria, and pollutants. Dairy, in fact, may be the most unhealthy food Americans routinely consume.[2]

Organic animal products produced by well-treated animals may be better. I hope cows who are "grass fed, poetry read, and tucked in bed" are happy cows, but even happy cows produce organic milk that is too high in protein, fat, cholesterol, pus, calories, and cow hormones. We could avoid some excess calories by sticking with low-fat dairy and egg whites, but then the concentration of animal protein is even higher. Unfortunately, the animal protein is just as unhealthy as the fat. In fact, after a lifetime of conducting original peer-reviewed research on the subject, Colin Campbell came to the conclusion that the protein in milk is "the most relevant [closely connected] chemical carcinogen ever identified."[3]

And we certainly do not need milk to get enough calcium. This is one of the best-funded myths in all of nutrition. Dairy consumption does not do the body good or even result in stronger bones. The *majority* (approximately 75 percent) of the world's population is lactose-intolerant, physically unable to properly digest milk (this includes about fifty million Americans).[4] Literally billions of people around the world grow strong and healthy without consuming *any* dairy (as I witnessed firsthand during my mission in Taiwan). We Americans, on the other hand, consume an enormous amount of dairy products, and yet we have one of the highest rates of osteoporosis (weak bones) in the world.[5] In fact, increased calcium intake does not protect against osteoporosis.[6] Calcium comes from the soil to us through plants, and the body tightly regulates its absorption. Consuming dairy and meat increases the acid level of the body and may cause the body to draw on stores of calcium and other minerals from the bones to neutralize the acid and bring the body back into proper pH balance. Thus animal food consumption can lead to a loss of the body's calcium.[7]

With all of the evidence against milk consumption, what keeps us from making a culture-wide dietary change? Sadly, it seems anti-American to not consume milk. We are often told that milk is nature's most perfect food. I used to think this way until others reminded me that it is not entirely "natural" for adult mammals to consume the secretions produced by another species for her young, especially well past the time we are weaned.[8] We no more need cow milk than we need cat or rat milk. Cow's milk is designed to help the newborn calf double in weight in 8 weeks and grow to over 600 pounds when weaned.[9] It is nature's most perfect food . . . for a baby cow. And yes, eggs are also a perfect food . . . for the unhatched chick.

Most WFPB experts agree that if they had to choose just one category of food Americans should eliminate from their diet, it would be dairy, in all its forms. Yes (oh so sadly!), this includes all 31 flavors of Baskin Robbins' ice cream. Now there is a food I wish were perfect!

If dairy and eggs are so unhealthy, why are they not specifically mentioned in the Word of Wisdom? One obvious answer is that not everything that is unhealthy or harmful to the body is specifically prohibited in the Word of Wisdom. Illicit drugs, for example, are nowhere mentioned, yet no one doubts that cocaine and heroin are more harmful than coffee or tea. In response to those who would excuse the use of illicit drugs because they are not specifically prohibited in the Word of Wisdom, President Gordon B. Hinckley stated:

> What a miserable excuse. There is likewise no mention [in the Word of Wisdom] of the hazards of diving into an empty swimming pool or of jumping from an overpass onto the freeway. But who doubts the deadly consequences of such? Common sense would dictate against such behavior.[10]

I believe once people understand the evidence against dairy and eggs, common sense will likewise dictate against their widespread consumption.

There is actually something glorious and sacred about the flesh of animals as well as the milk and eggs they produce. From a tiny egg emerges one of God's beautiful animal creations, a true miracle by any measure. Milk is the perfect vital nutrient created by the mother animal for her young. Animal flesh is the physical tabernacle for God's amazing creatures. Further, God has ordained and made it possible for humans to obtain nutrients from these creatures in times of need. But in normal times, we can easily get all the nutrients we need (and more) from plant foods without killing the animals or eating their eggs or drinking their milk; and since they are packaged with much that can harm the human body, there are no good nutritional reasons to consume them. Let's save them for times of famine.

# Real Mormons ❧ Real Stories

## *Tandi's Story*

My journey to a plant-based diet began when I was 22 years old. My daughter was about three months old at the time, and we were applying for life insurance. We had the usual blood tests required by the insurance company and were told we had to pay a higher premium for me because at age 22 my cholesterol level was 220! I couldn't believe it! I was a little overweight at the time, but overall I felt "normal" and healthy.

Then, over the course of the next five months I became very ill. I had very little energy and suffered horrible, debilitating joint pain and muscle pain. I had severe digestive problems, stomach cramping that would cause me to sweat because of the pain, and diarrhea so bad that there were times we would be a mile from home going to a store and would have to turn around and go home. I began to lose weight rapidly and went from about 110 to 89 lbs in a matter of a couple of months. My arms and legs felt heavy, and it was difficult for me to even raise my arm to feed my daughter in her high chair. I told my doctor that I felt like a 90-year-old woman.

I also suffered from severe infertility, polycystic ovarian syndrome, amenorrhea (complete lack of menstruation), and a laundry list of other health problems. I went through many, many tests. They did identify that I had an autoimmune disease as my Antinuclear Antibody Test was positive, but they just weren't sure what autoimmune disease I had. A long list of possibilities was given. There were days amid all the pain and fatigue when I thought I was going to die.

I started researching on my own because doctors could not give me any answers, and I had spent the last six months in and out of doctors' offices and countless hours in the hospital having test after test done. I began slowly changing my diet. My weight normalized within a few months, but the joint pain and fatigue still plagued me. The changes I made were pretty standard but not enough to fully recover: I removed red meat from my diet, ate organic meat and dairy and more whole grains, fruits, and vegetables. I improved and became functional, although I didn't have a lot of energy. Over the course of the next several years I had bouts of severe fatigue, pain, and heavy limbs that made it difficult to function for a few days to a week and then I would feel okay. Even though the severity eased up, I still suffered from infertility and amenorrhea, along with bouts of severe fatigue, pain, and difficulty functioning.

I finally started to connect the dots when I attended a nutrition class held by the Utah Valley State College community education program. It was a raw foods class. I had no idea what raw food was, but I was intrigued and wanted to learn all I could about nutrition. The instructor taught us that the milk of any species is only designed for its own baby and that an older child or adult had no need for mother's milk or the milk of any other species. Things just started to click for me, and I went home and threw out the cow's milk, cheese, and all other dairy products, along with all meat and eggs, and started on a plant-based diet immediately!

Within three months of removing all dairy, eggs, and meat from my diet I had more energy at 27 than I had ever had in my life, and I had my first period in over three years! I was thrilled. I did not suffer any longer from any joint pain, muscle aches, fatigue, or foggy thinking, and my female problems improved dramatically.

I purchased several books on the Word of Wisdom, including Dr. Christopher's *Just What Is the Word of Wisdom?* and I studied D&C 89 prayerfully. I realized that God had provided us the perfect blueprint for optimal health but unfortunately due to our "foolish traditions" surrounding food, we use the provisions given for times of famine or lack of adequate food as an excuse for our dietary excesses.

I have been on a plant-based diet now for nine years, and I am happy to report the improvements were permanent. I never had another bout of pain, fatigue or debility, and my fertility symptoms improved as well. I went back to school and obtained my bachelor's degree in health science and then completed the Certificate in Plant-Based Nutrition program from eCornell. I have now helped dozens of people suffering from a myriad of health problems, from type 2 diabetes to fibromyalgia, regain their health through a plant-based diet. When the Word of Wisdom is studied with an open heart and an open mind, and its precepts are implemented, healing is dramatic and miraculous. I am truly grateful for the knowledge I have gained over the last nine years, and I am so thankful to have regained my health!

*Tandi Hartle, age 36, lives in Eagle Mountain, Utah. She and her husband have two children, ages 14 and 11. Tandi earned her BS in Natural Health Science and has a Certificate in Plant-Based Nutrition from eCornell and a Nutritional Herbalist Certificate.*

# 6

# Science and the Word of Wisdom

In a 2004 paper published in the *Journal of the American Medical Association*, the authors reviewed data from epidemiological, clinical, and laboratory studies from 1980 to 2002 in order to "identify and quantify the leading causes of mortality in the United States."[1] Their results confirmed that the top three causes of death in America are

1. Tobacco use
2. Poor diet and physical inactivity
3. Alcohol consumption

It is reassuring to know that the three most significant causes of death in the United States are addressed in the Word of Wisdom and are each within our control!

As I've studied the WFPB literature, I'm amazed by the congruence between what these experts say science tells us about the optimal diet for our bodies and what the Word of Wisdom says. Here are the similarities:

1. Tobacco, alcohol, and drugs are harmful and should be avoided.
2. Plants are the optimal foods for our health and are best eaten in season.
3. Grains (starches) should be the staple of our diets.
4. Meat should be eaten rarely, if at all.

In addition, these experts also agree that

1. We need to get adequate sleep but not too much sleep. (D&C 88:124)
2. Occasional fasting is good for our health. (D&C 59:13–19)

There is less agreement among these experts on whether coffee is harmful, and there is no agreement about tea, especially green tea. So here, the Word of Wisdom gives Latter-day Saints the edge. While we certainly don't know all the reasons why, we do know we are better off not consuming coffee or tea.

Likewise, while plant-based diet experts agree that the bulk of the scientific data clearly concludes that the optimal human diet consists of whole plants, centered on grains, with little or no meat, there are certainly many other experts who disagree. In fact, the controversies on this topic are numerous. Fortunately, because of the Word of Wisdom, we don't need to wait for all the scientific evidence to come in before we decide what is best for our temporal well-being.

Science is extremely helpful, but scientific evidence is not enough to guide our lives. Even today there are those who maintain that science cannot "prove" a causal relationship between smoking and lung cancer. The fact is they are right. Given the reductionist standards for defining a "cause" in science, the complexity of the human body and its amazing ability to adapt and survive, and the lab conditions needed to obtain irrefutable proof that tobacco "causes" lung cancer, science will likely never determine this link beyond any doubt. Fortunately, because they had the Word of Wisdom, early Saints did not need to wait for science. Nor do we need to wait until science has established, beyond doubt, what the optimal diet for human beings is. We've already been told.

## Ancient Wisdom Still Unfolding

Historically, many people have understood, whether by tradition, religion, or personal experience, that whole-plant foods, with little or no meat, are optimal for the human body. Vegetarian diets are not a modern innovation. Based on the story in Genesis, Adam and Eve consumed a vegetarian diet in the Garden of Eden, and since that time various people and populations have chosen to abstain from consuming animal foods. The earliest and largest bodies of ancient texts advocating a vegetarian diet come from ancient India and Greece.[2] Various Asian religious sects, especially Hinduism, Buddhism, and Jainism have discouraged consuming animals. While most Christian traditions have not promoted a vegetarian diet, many well-known Christian leaders and believers did choose to abstain from eating animal flesh (for example, Origen, Leo Tolstoy, John Wesley, and Albert Schweitzer).[3]

While science is still working out the details for exactly why the body thrives best on a whole food, plant-based diet, the basic principles have been known for generations. Long before scientists had worked out the biochemistry for vitamins, minerals, protein, and fiber, wise mothers were telling their kids to eat their vegetables. Ironically, now that we have more evidence for the importance of vegetables than at any other time in history, some of our children (along with many of us adults) are eating *fewer* vegetables than some earlier generations. *More science does not equal more wisdom.*

Nevertheless, more and better science can be extremely valuable, and the science of nutrition has grown exponentially during the last two centuries. Notwithstanding, I'm discovering that much of the science I'm only now becoming acquainted with has actually been known for *decades.* In fact, I've been surprised to learn how clearly many early Church leaders and members have understood the relationship between diet and disease, including the potential hazards associated with consuming meats and refined foods. However, the truths they have known have always been mixed in with half-truths and untruths, just as it has been throughout history.

Thus, I believe the relationship between science and revelation has been critical to the ongoing unfolding of our collective and individual understanding of the Lord's will. The text of Section 89 may have been given to Joseph Smith in 1833, but the meaning of this text is still being revealed to us, "line upon line, precept upon precept" (2 Nephi 28:30). In my study of Church history, I find that Latter-day Saints consistently interpret the Word of Wisdom through the lens of contemporary science. While they also use the Word of Wisdom to evaluate the science, it seems impossible for us to read Section 89 completely outside the framework of the science, culture, and traditions that form our worldview. Thus, the relationship between science and the Word of Wisdom is a dialectical one.

Below, I will highlight just three of many past publications by LDS authors that illustrate this evolving dialectic. These publications illustrate how clearly Latter-day Saints have historically understood so many of the facts now established by science that support a whole food, plant-based diet, as well as how LDS authors have used the Word of Wisdom to interpret the science of their time and to sort out competing and contradictory claims. Perhaps because of the dialectic between the wisdom found in this revelation and the wisdom found in science, it should not be surprising that there is an ever-changing, diverse understanding of this revelation.

# 1937 — John and Leah Widtsoe

Elder John A. Widtsoe (apostle and distinguished scholar) and his accomplished wife, Leah D. Widtsoe (Church leader and prominent home economics educator), conducted the most thorough investigation of the relationship between the science of nutrition and the Word of Wisdom in their 1937 book, *The Word of Wisdom: A Modern Interpretation*.[4] In this carefully researched work (used as the LDS Church Priesthood study course in 1938), the Widtsoes attempt to show how science clarifies our understanding and confirms the teachings of the Word of Wisdom. Although the book was written over 75 years ago, the Widtsoes expound on almost every major point made by plant-based diet experts today. Here are some highlights:

- They document the decrease in "infectious diseases" (communicable diseases) along with the (already!) **alarming increase in "chronic or degenerative diseases"** (noncommunicable diseases), both in the general population and among the Latter-day Saints (p. 14).

- They use the current science to assert the **"growing consensus" that a lack of good nutrition is a primary cause for the prevalence of chronic illness** (cancer, diabetes, heart disease, kidney disease, etc.) (p. 18).

- They note the **tremendous economic strain caused by chronic illness** and substance abuse, suggesting, "the national debt could be wiped off quickly if the laws of health were fully understood and obeyed" (p. 22).

- They argue that **we need to pay as much attention to the things we should eat** (fruits, vegetables, grains) **as to the things we should not** (tobacco, alcohol, coffee, tea, etc.) (p. 21).

- They outline in great detail **the nutritive value of plant foods,** and assert that **"plants [contain] all of the necessary food substances:** Proteins (flesh-formers), fats, starches and other carbohydrates, minerals and water." They are also the best sources of vitamins (p. 126).

- They agree that **"grains, or cereals, were ordained to be 'the staff of life'** for human consumption" (p. 174).

- They explain why **"soft, highly refined and concentrated foods" are lacking in nutrition** and note that these foods are (already!) becoming too large a percent of the modern diet (p. 15).

- They detail **the health hazards of consuming meat** and admonish readers to **eat "plenty of fruit and vegetables, with grain foods and very little meat"** (p. 81).
- They assert, **"Natural foods, as prepared by Mother Nature, are best for man** and beast. Beware of all artificial synthetic food products or drinks made by man for commercial gain" (p. 228).
- They warn us to **not believe "all that is told by shrewd advertising"** by "conspiring men in the last days" who are "far more interested in their own pocket-book than in the public health" (p. 230).

Throughout the book, the Widtsoes delight in pointing out the numerous ways modern science confirms and supports the Word of Wisdom. At the same time, they question why it is that with all the knowledge about health that we Latter-day Saints possess, we are not a healthier people. They conclude:

> The answer is obvious: It is evident that people of the Church are not observing fully all the factors of health as given in the Word of Wisdom. . . . One can not say that to refrain from smoking and from drinking tea, coffee or alcohol is to keep fully the Word of Wisdom. . . . The many "do's" in the inspired document are as important as the "don't's." Unquestionably, the Word of Wisdom is not lived completely or the people would receive a greater fullness of the promised reward—a long life of physical health, while the destroying angel of sickness and death would pass by and not slay them. (pp. 20–21)

While the Widtsoes did not advocate a 100 percent vegetarian diet, it appears the reason they did not is that the science of their time was still very prejudiced in favor of meat consumption and had not even begun to question the wisdom of dairy and eggs. Science had not yet verified, beyond reasonable doubt, that all animal foods are completely unnecessary for optimal human health. Nevertheless, the Widtsoes assert:

- "The old doctrine that meat is peculiarly able to endow men with strength, endurance and courage has long been shown to be fallacious. Vegetarians have often excelled in competitive sports" (p. 212).
- Meat proteins are more expensive/wasteful than vegetable proteins (p. 212).
- "All of the necessary food constituents are found in plants. From that point of view, vegetarianism should be practicable. . . . The

possibility of subsisting wholly on non-animal products cannot be denied" (p. 136).

- "Many vegetarians have lived well and happily to a ripe old age" (p. 136).
- "Meat should, indeed, form a minor part of the human dietary" (p. 218).

In everything they wrote, the Widtsoes try to stay close to both the meaning of the Word of Wisdom and the science of their day, readily admitting that science would continue to progress, while believing the best of science would never contradict the word of God. They wrote:

> Scientific knowledge concerning man's diet is yet in its infancy. Many new angles to old truths are constantly being discovered. When such are definitely established in the best laboratories of nutrition to be facts, not mere theories, then they may be accepted and used, and they will be found to be in harmony with the general principles set forth by the Word of Wisdom. (p. 233)

Now that the science of nutrition has concluded that a purely plant-based diet is viable for all life stages and activity levels,[5] I am confident that if the Widtsoes were writing today, they would undoubtedly endorse such a diet for those wishing to adhere to a more healthy lifestyle. In fact, when they revised their book for publication in 1950, they were much more direct about the value of moving away from meat consumption in times other than winter and cold.[6]

Scientific evidence notwithstanding, it takes a very long time even for scientists, much less the general population, to fully understand and appreciate, let alone implement, the best knowledge available. The Widtsoes use the example of meat both to show how inspired the Word of Wisdom is and how prejudices to the contrary are slow to change. They state:

> At the time that the Word of Wisdom was given, meat, when it could be obtained, was largely used by all classes. It was generally looked upon as the best and most necessary food for full health. Those who raised their voices in opposition to this view were held to be fanatical, untrustworthy "food faddists." Alas! Some people hold that opinion today!

> It was therefore a courageous departure from accepted
> practice to teach that meat should be used "sparingly," and
> further to suggest that man may live without meat as implied
> in the words, "they should not be used, only in times of win-
> ter, or of cold or famine." (p. 217)

Since the 1950s, the evidence that animal foods are not optimal for
the human body has continued to grow. Notwithstanding the amount
of evidence that has accumulated, the Widtsoes would have been astonished to learn that most Latter-day Saints today are as prejudiced in
favor of meat as they were in the Widtsoes' day. Although much of the
science the Widtsoes outline in their book is now dated, their primary
claims have been verified by further research, and yet the average diet in
America today is arguably *less* healthy. *Increased knowledge does not equal
increased wisdom.*

# 1969 — Ray G. Cowley, MD

In 1969, Dr. Ray Cowley, an LDS medical doctor, referred to the Word
of Wisdom as "An 1833 Guide for the Prevention of Heart Disease."
This was the title of the article he published that year in the official
Church magazine, *Improvement Era.*[7] In reading it, I was struck by how
contemporary it felt even though it was written *over 40 years ago.* I had
assumed it was only recently that we fully understood the intimate relationship between diet and heart disease. Why would by-pass surgery
be such a large industry today if we had known for so long that heart
disease is preventable through good diet? Yet in this article, Dr. Cowley presents study after study that clearly link diet to the number one
killer in America and refers to hundreds more studies that demonstrate
how this disease is associated with "greater consumption of animal protein, saturated fat, refined carbohydrates, and the decreased use of cereal
grains" (p. 63). Despite the evidence, the same prejudices that existed
when the Widtsoes were writing in the 1930s persisted in the 1960s.
Cowley writes:

> Although this relationship is now supported by almost in-
> controvertible proof, the medical profession has been slow to
> accept findings that decimate a long-standing and traditional
> medical dictum that a steady and large dietary intake of an-
> imal or fowl origin meat is essential to good health. (p. 63)

After reviewing the scientific evidence and marveling at how clearly the Word of Wisdom admonishes us to eat "little or no meat," Dr. Cowley concludes:

> The only conceivable explanation for Section 89 of the Doctrine and Covenants is that it came from a highly advanced and infallible source of intelligence beyond this earth. The contents of this section should be carefully studied, and personal eating and living habits should be formulated on the basis of advice given therein, for this is of a certainty a divinely inspired guide to good health and long life, with transcendent rewards for compliance that should induce the most skeptical to put it to an honest test. (p. 63)

Of course Church leaders have always agreed with Dr. Cowley's assessment of the divine origin of this health code. In the 1998 general conference, for example, President Gordon B. Hinckley said:

> I regard [the Word of Wisdom] as the most remarkable document on health of which I know. It came to the Prophet Joseph Smith in 1833, when relatively little was known of dietary matters. Now the greater the scientific research, the more certain becomes the proof of Word of Wisdom principles.[8]

# 1993 — Kenneth E. Johnson, MD

In 1993, Dr. Kenneth Johnson published *The Word of Wisdom Food Plan: A Medical Review of the Mormon Doctrine*, a book supporting a WFPB diet.[9] The way I discovered this book is interesting. My good friend, Abbie Kim, was working as an RN in the rehabilitation unit of the Utah Valley Regional Medical Center, where they regularly care for patients suffering from heart disease and stroke. Of course family members are often there to care for their loved ones, and one day the wife of one stroke patient was using Dr. Johnson's book to encourage her husband to improve his diet and survive his illness. She herself was following a WFPB diet and was trim and healthy, but her family was not. She was discouraged by their poor health and unwillingness to change their diet and was very eager to share the book with anyone who would listen. When she learned that Abbie is Korean, she was overjoyed and excitedly shared with her something she had found in the book about the Korean War.

In the book, Dr. Johnson records the following study, related to his experience as a member of the Army Medical Corps stationed in Korea during the 1950–53 Korean War. He writes:

> In autopsies of the soldiers who died, the difference between the American and Korean soldiers was very apparent.
>
> Autopsy studies on Korean soldiers showed no evidence of early atherosclerosis, the beginning of heart disease. They were protected from the ravages of atherosclerosis by their plant-centered diet, low in fat and cholesterol. But [90 percent of] the young American soldiers showed early evidence of the disease; in fact, the disease was far advanced in some of them. (p. 29)

Sadly, this fine LDS doctor did not consume the same "plant-centered diet" that protected the arteries of the Korean soldiers. He had to suffer two heart attacks and two open-heart multiple by-pass surgeries before finally discovering a "new" diet that would arrest the disease. What was this "new diet"? None other than the one revealed to the Prophet Joseph Smith over 150 years earlier. If he had only better understood and kept the Word of Wisdom from his youth, he could have avoided that fate.

Not wanting others to go through what he did, Dr. Johnson produced a book that presents in sufficient detail all the explanation necessary to help his fellow Latter-day Saints better understand and appreciate the marvelous counsel given in the Word of Wisdom. The science he presents is far in advance of what the Widtsoes, and even Dr. Cowley, had available to them, but the basic principles are the same. The main difference is that Dr. Johnson now had greater scientific backing to support and encourage a fully plant-based diet. He writes:

> We know now that the food plan for optimum health and the prevention of premature death should derive about 10 percent of its calories from fat, about 10 percent from protein and 80 percent from complex carbohydrates. These calories are best supplied by grains, rice, potatoes, legumes, fruits and vegetables. Few or no calories should come from flesh (products of meat, eggs and milk). (p. 104)

Dr. Johnson's confidence is bolstered not just by science but by numerous other doctors who by then had had many years of experience assisting *thousands* of patients in overcoming serious chronic illness by switching to a plant-centered diet. He writes:

Scattered among the numerous diets that consistently fail are several medically-sound diets that follow the tenets of the Word of Wisdom.

These are plant-centered, with emphasis on complex carbohydrates, limits on protein, and severe limits on fat. (p. 95)

The authors of the diets Dr. Johnson cites as "medically-sound" are among the many I have encountered since I began my own plant-centered journey in 2011: Nathan Pritikin; John McDougall, MD; Dean Ornish, MD; and Neal Barnard, MD. There are many more experts who could be added to this list including Caldwell Esselstyn, MD; Colin Campbell, PhD; Hans Diehl, PhD; and Joel Fuhrman, MD. These are but a few of the many who have demonstrated that the diet revealed through Joseph Smith in 1833 can and does help people obtain their optimal health.

## This Revelation Continues to be Revealed

As I've said, I keep being surprised at how long we have "known" the nutritional truths I've been learning. It is now evident that nothing in the Word of Wisdom was actually new even in Joseph Smith's day. All the nutrition counsel it contains can be found among the recommendations of his time.[10] Indeed, all the nutrition counsel in Section 89 has been known for centuries, possibly millennia. It makes sense that something as fundamental as what to eat to have strong and healthy bodies would be wisdom sought out, practiced, and passed down through generations of time.

The Word of Wisdom is unique not because of *what* it recommends but because of *Who* recommends it—and because it has withstood the test of time. While the wisdom it contains had been known to previous generations, just as today, this wisdom has always been mixed in with falsehoods, superstitions, and confusing half-truths.[11] There is not now, just as there has never been, a consensus among experts as to the optimal diet for human beings.

In every detailed analysis of the Word of Wisdom ever written by Church leaders or members, it is apparent they used their understanding of science and nutrition to interpret the Word of Wisdom. No one takes the wording at face value; they all bring their presuppositions to the text (as have I). Our collective understanding and appreciation of the Word of Wisdom will continue to evolve over time, along with the scientific conclusions. This is how this revelation can contain ancient wisdom and, at the same time, "will *yet* reveal many great and important things pertaining to the Kingdom of God" (Articles of Faith 9, emphasis added).

Perhaps, then, it should not be surprising to find that *my* understanding and appreciation of these words of wisdom is also evolving over time and that it has taken scientific evidence for me to more fully comprehend a revelation I've known since youth. And because science and our understanding continue to evolve, I must assume that at least some of what I now believe will need to change in the future; some of my claims will become outdated, and some may need to be abandoned completely.

As it is with many revelations, we are usually much better at understanding what we should *do* in light of the revelation than we are at trying to *explain why* the Lord told us to do it. In fact our explanations can create stumbling blocks when they turn out to be incorrect. Of course, cutting-edge science can reveal new insights into God's revelations, but science will never give us all the reasons why we need to obey God's commandments. As the Prophet Joseph Smith said, we probably will not know all the reasons until long *after* we have obeyed. He writes:

> This is the principle on which the government of heaven is conducted—by revelation adapted to the circumstances in which the children of the kingdom are placed. Whatever God requires is right, no matter what it is, although we may not see the reason thereof till long after the events transpire.
> . . . Blessings offered, but rejected, are no longer blessings, but become like the talent hid in the earth by the wicked and slothful servant.[12]

Note how God's commandments are "adapted to the circumstances in which the children of the kingdom are placed." I think this is certainly true of the Word of Wisdom, which appears to be adapted specifically for our modern-day circumstances. When in history have we needed this counsel more? Peoples in former times ate whatever was available; they rarely had much choice. We do.

## Word of Wisdom Truths from Non-Mormons

Interestingly, non-LDS scientists and other experts are the ones finally awakening the world to the power of a Word of Wisdom diet. This message is so important that God appears to be revealing these truths through multiple channels, including both revelation and advances in science, to peoples of all religions. After all, Mormons are not the only ones in need of this precious wisdom.

While it is true that the Word of Wisdom gives the Latter-day Saints tremendous health advantages, many Mormons would be surprised to learn that we are probably not the single healthiest population in America. Seventh-day Adventists hold the distinction of being among the few longest-lived populations in the world.[13] Like Latter-day Saints, Adventists have what they consider to be revelations on diet and health, which, interestingly, were received about 30 years after Joseph Smith received the revelation on the Word of Wisdom. Like the Word of Wisdom, these Adventist revelations led the way well before science confirmed their truths. Because of these revelations, Adventists do not consume alcohol or tobacco. Tea and coffee are discouraged, but in addition, they also discourage the consumption of meat. Instead, they emphasize eating fresh whole-plant foods. Approximately 35 percent of Adventists are vegetarians.[14] LDS scholar Hugh Nibley notes, "on the whole the Seventh Day Adventists are better keepers of the Word of Wisdom than we are."[15]

A short time after discovering the whole food, plant-based diet, I was searching for like-minded people in Utah and quickly discovered that many Seventh-day Adventists are prominent in promoting this lifestyle. I had an opportunity to talk with two different Adventists. On both occasions, the person I spoke with said the same thing, "We feel God gave Adventists a truth, so we have an obligation to share that truth with others." They view the knowledge they have as something precious, and they do, in fact, actively share their dietary truths with people not of their faith. For example, they regularly sponsor events to share the benefits of a plant-based diet with people who are not Adventists; they do this not for the purpose of converting people to their religion, but to help others understand the connection between diet and health. How many of us feel so grateful for the wisdom found in D&C 89 that we enthusiastically seek to share it with others not of our faith?

I recently ran across a discussion on a non-LDS forum on the Internet. When someone referenced Mormons and the Word of Wisdom, a non-member stated that she lives in a town with a large LDS population but finds that most of the Mormons she knows "do not eat very healthfully." She was surprised to learn about the Word of Wisdom and said, "I need to bring this up to my [Mormon] friend. She may find it helpful. I have been trying to encourage her to go vegetarian but to no avail. . . . Maybe that will be the thing that helps her." I am not sure whether to be excited or disappointed at the thought of non-members teaching us the Word of Wisdom!

# Real Mormons ❧ Real Stories

## *Paul's Story*

My wife and I have always tried to eat with a mind toward health. But I enjoyed a good hamburger, barbequed tri-tips, chocolate shakes, ice cream, etc. In fact I would have been perfectly happy to have hamburgers for every meal. I still would—but I can't do it, because I know too much about what that would do to my body, not to mention the cows' bodies.

So my journey toward a plant-based diet came slowly. As my wife became totally plant-based, I supported her (easy to do since she looks amazing at 57). We had mostly plant-based food at home, except for cheese and a few other things like that. She learned to cook meals that could be done completely plant-based or with a little bit of cheese or even meat thrown in.

At 46 I was in very good health, or so I thought. I was in a kickboxing class, could do 80 pushups, and could run forever. But my feet started to tingle a lot. The tingling gradually grew into outright pain. Terrible, unbearable pain. I went to several doctors who simply couldn't figure out what was going on. When they took x-rays of my feet they were astounded. My bones were disappearing. I was osteoporotic as an otherwise healthy 46-year-old male: practically unheard of.

After numerous tests, they discovered my kidneys were throwing out all of my calcium, causing my parathyroid glands to grab the calcium from my bones so that my body would have enough to function. The docs gave me prescriptions to help my condition. Nothing worked and the meds had weird, unacceptable side effects. During this time they also discovered I was pre-diabetic, glucose intolerant. Apparently my feet found out I was about to become diabetic and decided to get peripheral neuropathy early—thus the tingling, numbness and sharp pains in my feet. (I realize that numbness and pain don't seem too congruent, but just ask anybody with neuropathy about that. They won't be able to explain why, but they'll make a pretty convincing case that it happens.)

So now I had two problems: diabetes and the kidney thing. I had also had two very bad kidney stones, requiring three surgeries between them because they would not pass on their own. I was given more medicine for the diabetes issue and was told to cut way down on carbs: go easy on the fruit and bread and eat meat. My wife was very supportive and went out of her way to make sure I could follow the standard American diet for diabetes.

But nothing worked. My blood sugars were high (although not outrageous since I was only pre-diabetic, not full-on diabetic), and my kidneys were still throwing out my calcium—plus I was growing a third arm from the meds (just kidding—but I really didn't like the meds). I also got high blood pressure. My wife suggested I try going totally vegan. I resisted at first, but she said, "You can do this for three months, and if it doesn't work, go back to your animal products." I decided I could do almost anything for three months, so I took her up on the challenge.

I went to my doctor and had her run all the blood and urine tests on me to have as a baseline. She told me I was crazy, but she went along with the plan. Then I went completely one hundred percent plant-based for three months and had her run those same tests again. I will never forget the doctor's appointment when she discussed the test results with me. She walked into the room and said, "Well Paul, you should have gone to medical school instead of law school. You have cured yourself." All of my numbers were completely normal. I thought, "Dang it, there go the hamburgers." I wasn't necessarily happy, but I was relieved to know there was actually a cure that would work for me.

Since then I have had long periods of eating completely plant-based and long periods where I ate mostly plant-based (90-95%). I am still tempted by meat and cheese but I will never go back to eating the way I used to. There is not a single animal protein to be found in our house, except for the dog, and we're not too keen on the idea of eating her. I am utterly convinced that a plant-based diet is the healthiest way to live, and for me, it's life saving. I could not have continued on with the health problems I was having and had any kind of life. My feet still hurt due to irreversible nerve damage, but the only meds I am on are a couple that calm the nerves enough that I can tolerate the pain. I have learned to ignore it and have a pretty normal, happy life.

My life experience has led me to the undeniable conclusion that someone really knew what he was doing when he wrote Section 89. It's high time for members of the LDS faith to take their Word of Wisdom compliance to the next level.

*Paul Johnson, 61, lives in Orem, Utah. He and his wife, Orva, are the parents of nine children. They are expecting their 30th grandchild. Paul is an attorney. When not visiting grandkids, he enjoys exploring the mountains of Utah and likes fast cars and shooting handguns.*

You can find the story of Paul's wife, Orva Johnson, in Appendix One: *More* Real Mormons ✻ Real Stories.

# 7

# Common Objections

I have to confess: before I started to eat this way, I could not imagine giving up animal foods or eliminating most processed foods. Just the year before changing my diet a doctor had suggested to my mother that she stop using milk. I remember thinking, "You have got to be CRAZY! How is that even possible?" So, I completely understand the objections people make to this diet. In this chapter, I'll address a few of them.

## Why Aren't We Taught These Things?

If it is so clear what we should and should not be eating, why haven't all the experts who write about nutrition and are constantly interviewed by the media made that plain? Why doesn't the US Department of Agriculture (USDA) promote a strictly plant-based diet? If a WFPB diet truly were the answer to chronic disease, wouldn't my doctor have told me?

Of course, all of us have already been told much more about good health and nutrition than most of us bother to use. We all know we should eat more fruits and vegetables, get more exercise, and cut back on soda and junk foods. Even children know Krispy Kreme doughnuts are not health foods. But how many Americans do what they already know is right? Perhaps one reason we may not have heard the WFPB message is that we don't fully embrace even the health advice we've been given.

But there are other reasons we don't hear much about the benefits of a WFPB diet. The fact is it takes money to promote a message. It takes money to not only educate the common person on the street, but also to educate doctors, the government, and even PhDs in nutrition. Who has the money to fund this education? Unfortunately, the people who have the money are the very people who have a financial interest in promoting a diet that is the opposite of a WFPB diet. The people with the money are the people making a profit selling a diet heavy in meat, dairy, and highly processed junk foods. Guess who is getting their message out?

A critical key to understanding the confusion about good nutrition is the plain fact that there is very little money to be made in promoting a truly healthy diet. Relatively few business people get rich by selling only whole foods. On the other hand, I can think of several multi-billion dollar food conglomerations that might go out of business if everyone ate like I eat. Ironically, even the medical establishment thrives on our being sick. Certainly pharmaceutical companies do.

How many commercials do you see on TV promoting asparagus, strawberries, kidney beans, or whole wheat? Compare that to the number of commercials that promote dairy, refined foods and beverages, and restaurants serving the standard American diet. Even with all the scary disclaimers, the pharmaceutical companies have much more ability to get their message out than do all the fruit and vegetable farmers of the world. There are only so many fortunes to be made off of broccoli or cauliflower. Food executives know that "selling unprocessed or minimally processed whole foods will always be a fool's game."[1] The more you process whole foods, the more money you can make off of them. You can't patent bananas or cucumbers, but you can patent processed foods and the drugs you can sell to people who get sick on them.[2]

We consumers ultimately decide what products we will buy, and food corporations can't exist unless they produce what we want. But what we want is often more influenced by the biology of our brains than our ability to reason. Like all animals, we are biologically adapted to seek substances that stimulate pleasure signals in our brains. Fortunately, the most harmful drugs are illegal, but there are plenty of legal stimulants to choose from, including nicotine and alcohol. And now science is uncovering the unpleasant fact that foods rich in sugar and fat, though certainly not as harmful as illegal drugs, are physically addictive through precisely the same biological mechanisms. Like drugs, we are finding that sugary sweets, high-fat foods, and even meat and cheese stimulate an increased release of dopamine, the brain's primary pleasure-producing chemical. Not only does this mechanism produce immediate pleasure, we are biologically disposed to seek more of it. Like drugs, these foods can habituate us to the rush of dopamine and strengthen our desire to consume them, and like drugs, we may find we have to consume them in increasing quantities to compensate for the diminishing rewards we experience over time.[3]

When we say we can't give up meat, cheese, sweets, or junk foods, it may be true that we can't give them up without some degree of discomfort or even withdrawal. We have become so adapted to the pleasure signals they produce in our bodies that we feel driven to consume them, despite the harm they are doing. Rats will choose cocaine over food, even to the point of their own starvation. They will likewise ignore healthy food when junk food is available to gorge themselves on.[4]

As moral agents, we certainly have the ability to resist indulging in these substances, but the combination of the pleasure they produce and their ready availability makes abuse easy. It should not surprise us that substance abuse is rampant in our society. As far as nicotine and alcohol are concerned, the government tries to protect us by regulating advertising, restricting access, and launching educational campaigns. While the government also tries to educate us on the dangers of diets high in simple sugars, cholesterol, and fats, they simultaneously subsidize the companies producing these very products and even aid in their marketing campaigns. Because we are biologically adapted to seek and consume high caloric food, in the war of mixed messages, we too often allow our biological drives to get the upper hand.

Even when we are not addicted to the worst junk foods, we tend to over consume food that is high in sugar, salt, and fat. This is true despite the fact that our bodies are biologically designed to eat the right amount of food to maintain perfect weight. Wild animals, even when they are in a naturally food-rich environment, eat only the amount of food they need to maintain proper weight, but we humans continually over consume food. Why? When the foods we consume are *un*naturally rich and calorically dense, our natural biological feedback systems are unable to fully cope, and our biological ability to sense how many calories we've consumed does not work efficiently.[5] Lab (and domesticated) animals will over-consume unnaturally rich food to the point of obesity, if given ready access to it. This food is not designed for human health; it is designed to tap into our biological drives and get us to want more of it.

The processed food corporations of the world know their food science well. They know how to manipulate the fat, sugar, and salt content of foods to sell products and create repeat customers.[6] Of course, we as consumers have a choice, and if we purchased only healthy foods, that is what we'd be offered. Fortunately, there is increasing demand for health food, and the food industry's incredible talents have produced some amazing products that are healthier. But if we only ate what is good for us, many companies, even many health food companies, would go out of business because *health is in whole foods, but the profit is in processing.* Sadly, companies producing harmful foods are in no danger of going under. We Americans, and now increasingly the rest of the world, are easily persuaded to pay for and consume a very large amount of what is not good for us.

How should we feel about a food system that produces products that sabotage our health and gets us to pay for it? Could the situation really be that dire? Interestingly, the introduction to Section 89 indicates the Lord knew exactly the situation we would be in and was preparing us with these words of wisdom:

> Behold, verily, thus saith the Lord unto you: In consequence of evils and designs which do and will exist in the hearts of conspiring men in the last days, I have warned you, and forewarn you, by giving unto you this word of wisdom by revelation. (D&C 89:4)

With so many powerful forces in our society enticing us to buy and consume products that are detrimental to our bodies, it is no wonder the Lord had to warn and forewarn us.

If we question why the field of nutrition is so rife with contradiction and confusion, we need to remember the power of money to distort truth. The same USDA that is commissioned to tell us what is best to eat is also responsible for supporting America's meat, dairy, and refined food industries. Do you think any amount of "scientific evidence" is going to be more powerful than the tremendous lobbying might of these huge businesses whose very lifeblood depends on our consuming their unhealthy products?

It is very hard to hear the health message of the Word of Wisdom when the marketing messages are better funded, exponentially louder, and more ubiquitous. When we believe the following myths, it is because it is in someone's financial interest that we do so:

- We need to eat meat to get adequate protein
- Eggs are an "ideal protein."
- Milk is good for our bones.
- Carbs are dangerous.
- We need more "healthy fats" in our diet.
- Olive oil, fish oil, and coconut oil are "health foods."
- It can't be wrong if everyone is doing it.

- If something is labeled "natural" it is good for you.
- Junk food is fun, popular, and will make you happy.
- Eating whatever foods you find delicious is part of the good life.
- Serving people rich, scrumptious foods shows you love them.

If it were easy to see through these messages, the Lord would not have needed to warn us. But to hear His message, we have to turn off the TV and listen to the still, small voice in Section 89.

## What about All the Experts Who Disagree?

I am persuaded that the bulk of scientific evidence clearly supports a low-fat whole food, plant-based diet, but not everyone is. There are plenty of experts who promote diets high in protein, fat, meat, and/or dairy. We are constantly bombarded by contradictory health claims, all supposedly backed by the "best science," to the point where most of us have given up trying to make sense of it all.

Many experts (including the USDA and many in the field of nutrition) say science supports a diet that includes refined foods, meat, and other animal products. They tell us junk food is fine in moderation. If you follow the guidelines produced by the USDA and still suffer from heart disease, diabetes, stroke, or many other preventable chronic illnesses, they blame it on factors beyond food, like genetics, lack of exercise, or the environment. Even if they believe there is a healthier diet, they don't believe people can stick to it, so they don't bother promoting it.

There are other experts who claim science promotes a diet very high in protein, who encourage consuming even more animal foods than the already high average Americans consume today.[7] There are even experts who believe "the science is clear" that the fewer carbohydrates we consume the better and that we cannot consume too much of the "right fats." Some of these experts believe fatty meat, lard, butter, and coconut oil are "health foods."[8]

There are also those who promote a totally "raw diet," consisting of raw vegetables, fruits, seeds, nuts, and "green smoothies."[9] I love green smoothies and raw foods, but as good as some vegetarian diets are, grains and other starches often play a very small role, if any, in these diets while the percent of calories from fats can be quite high. There must be a reason why the Lord tells us that grains are "good" and are, in fact, the "staff of life" (D&C 89:14, 16). Without starchy foods, it is very hard to get enough calories on a plant-based diet unless one adds a large amount of high-fat foods like nuts, seeds, and oils. In small quantities, these foods range from healthful to relatively harmless, but as the percentage of fat in our diet increases, so do various physical problems, including, of course, weight gain.[10]

For each diet, proponents have amassed a very tall stack of purported scientific evidence that supposedly confirms the efficacy of that diet. They have also collected testimonials from hundreds of patients whose health has been "turned around" on that diet. They can cite epidemiological and clinical studies all pointing to the same conclusion. Each is sure they are right.

Why the confusion? One key is noticing how each of these diets incorporates some food choices that are at least somewhat in harmony with a Word of Wisdom diet:

- Eating more fruits, vegetables, and/or green leafy vegetables.
- Using fresh, locally produced plant foods "in season."
- Eliminating/reducing animal foods or moving toward free-range, more naturally nourished animals for meat and animal products.
- Cutting down on fat, or at least using better fats.
- Eliminating highly refined foods, sometimes including vegetable oils.
- Eliminating dairy.
- Eliminating tobacco and at least reducing alcohol, coffee, and other stimulants.
- Eating more whole, unprocessed foods.
- Reducing the amount of junk food, sugar, and/or salt.

I believe most people promoting the variety of diets that only partially support the Word of Wisdom are doing so out of a sincere belief that they have found the optimal diet. For the most part, they seem motivated by the desire to help others. Further, I believe many of them are helping others develop better health: most diets are somewhat successful in helping people lose weight, at least initially, and this alone can account for many positive changes. In addition, our Standard American Diet (SAD) is so unhealthy that a switch to almost any other diet could easily result in tremendous health benefits. But all the evidence in the world that suggests a particular diet is *better* than SAD is not evidence that the diet is *optimal* for human health.

There are many reasons why even objective scientists find it difficult to speak with a unified voice on the subject of nutrition. First, the human body is complex and has an amazing ability to survive and even thrive on a variety of diets over long periods of time. Our bodies are built that way. We are also unable to do the controlled experiments on humans that we do on the physical world, man-made objects, or even animals; for example, we cannot totally isolate and control a single variable in humans. In addition, it is extremely difficult, expensive, and logistically impossible to conduct the type of *long-term* studies required to definitively nail down each nutrition fact.

But perhaps even more fundamental is the underlying approach modern science takes toward research. Modern science privileges reductionism (believing the whole can be understood in terms of its parts) over holistic thinking (believing the whole is *greater* than the sum of its parts). Most studies focus on tiny slices of human biology, divorced from the context of the greater whole. This type of research inevitably results in seemingly contradictory results.[11] Reductionism certainly has value in the study of biology, but reductionist thinking is best suited for machines, where the whole is a sum of the parts. Biological systems are not like machines, and the human body is more than biology: the mind and body and spirit are all intertwined, and our souls are interconnected with the rest of the universe. These are just a few of the reasons we probably should not wait until all the experts agree before we decide what to eat for our next meal.

Of course, all of this confusion does NOT mean that there is no consensus in the science of nutrition. Again, I am persuaded that the *bulk* of the scientific data *clearly* supports a low-fat whole food, plant-based diet, but I am not at all surprised there are many who disagree and who feel they have the scientific evidence to "prove it." They may have excellent reasons for their beliefs, but we have the Word of Wisdom to help us sort fact from fiction.

## What about Supplements and Other Health Products?

I am astonished when I recall the amount of time and energy I have expended throughout my life searching for the "right" products to solve various health issues. When I look around me, I see others expending the same time and energy in this never-ending search for solutions to serious health problems or to simply figure out how to feel better and have more energy. It should not be surprising to learn that this quest is not new to our day. Historically, people with time and money have always sought for foods, products, and procedures with special health claims (like Fountains of Youth). We usually take our health for granted, but when we have lost it, we suddenly have no greater priority.

Of course, the Word of Wisdom does not appear to be a guide to remedies for specific health problems. It does not provide counsel on how to treat health issues that may occur even after we are strictly following its counsel. *If someone is following a Word of Wisdom diet and still has health problems, what to do is beyond the scope of this book.* My focus is on those of us (perhaps the vast majority of us) who chase after all kinds of health answers before we've accepted and put into practice the counsel the Lord has already given us.

With the plethora of "wonder cures" on the Internet today, you'd think we could have solved all our critical health issues. Most of us (including me!) infinitely prefer an easy solution to a difficult one, even if the easy solution is more expensive. Vitamins and other supplements, medicinal herbs, essential oils, mineral water, energy bars, protein shakes, carb blockers, or fat burners may all have some valuable use, but I love the fact that the Word of Wisdom does not mention any of them. Instead, we are told to consume real food: wholesome plants in their season and animal flesh in times of need.

Where do all the nutrients in health supplements come from? They come from the earth, and God prepared the perfect way for these nutrients to get into our bodies: wholesome plants. As plants grow, they naturally embody a bewildering synthesis of amazing properties. As Michael Pollan explains:

> ...even the simplest food is a hopelessly complicated thing to analyze, a virtual wilderness of chemical compounds, many of which exist in intricate and dynamic relation to one another, and all of which together are in the process of changing from one state to another.[12]

Our bodies are designed to draw the nutrients they need from whole plants. It is an intricate and complex process that scientists are just beginning to understand. If you had to consciously tell your body what to do with each molecule of the plants you ingested, how far would you get? It might surprise you to know that even the most knowledgeable experts would not get much farther than you (at least relative to the enormity of the task). The effort, as Colin Campbell explains, is simply too complex:

> Every apple contains thousands of antioxidants whose names, beyond a few like vitamin C, are unfamiliar to us, and each of these powerful chemicals has the potential to play an important role in supporting our health. They impact thousands

upon thousands of metabolic reactions inside the human body. But calculating the specific influence of each of these chemicals isn't nearly sufficient to explain the effect of the apple as a whole. Because almost every chemical can affect every other chemical, there is an almost infinite number of possible biological consequences. And that's just from an apple.[13]

Where mortal minds can't comprehend, our bodies are supreme masters; our bodies know just what to do with the complex molecules of the wholesome plants we eat. But when we take these same whole plant foods and break their elements apart, process and refine them, and recombine them according to our limited understanding of how things work, we can sell them at a higher price, but it is unlikely we have improved on God's work. Our bodies are not designed to consume so-called health products; they are designed to consume whole foods. As we consume wholesome plants, we interact with the elements of the earth in the form our bodies have evolved to process. When given this nutritional support, our bodies are superbly designed to handle most of the health challenges sent their way.[14]

No doubt some health products are useful. Even if we only believe they can help, many otherwise useless products can have a strong impact on our health. Placebo effects are "genuine psychobiological events" that can have meaningful and long-lasting impact.[15] Beliefs are powerful, and what we believe about the world may have as much impact on our health as any health product or food we consume.[16] Beyond that, I believe there are many paths that can lead to improved health. God is very generous; surely He is willing to bless us in any number of ways, and our bodies seem to respond to many modalities.

But there does seem to be a danger in pinning our hopes on products and procedures: it leads us to believe we can forego the harder work of fundamentally changing our diet or lifestyle. Even if tiny amounts of expensive products have a positive impact on our health, how likely is it that these benefits would consistently outweigh the impact of consuming four to five pounds of nutrient-poor, processed and animal foods day in and day out?

The allure of the "easy fix" also leaves us susceptible to a cacophony of health claims from people who stand to profit from our desire to feel better. Sadly, what was true in the Widtsoes' day is even more true today: it is in too many people's financial interest to keep us confused so they can sell us products that are better for their pocketbooks than for our health.

Of course most of the people peddling health products are good people. Many of them may even have the best of intentions. I don't doubt that some of their products may be very useful under certain conditions, but does it make sense that our *daily* health would depend on expensive products that must be special ordered or on hi-tech gadgets that have only become available during the last fifty years?

Unfortunately, the natural health industry seems plagued with some of the same problems that the pharmaceutical industry is plagued with:

- Neither can make enough profit by selling us nutrients the way God designed them to be consumed (in the whole food).
- In order to make a good profit, both must find ways to improve on God's work, a work that has evolved over millions of years into a spectacularly complex system that is far beyond our present (or near-term) ability to comprehend.
- Both are willing to use poorly-executed research to promote their products and hide findings that are detrimental to their cause.
- Neither understands the human body well enough to anticipate the full effect (or side effects) of the products they recommend.

The same reductionist thinking that drives the pharmaceutical industries is all too evident in the natural, even holistic, health product industries. As Colin Campbell explains:

> The natural health community has also fallen prey to the ideology that chemicals ripped from their natural context are as good as or better than whole foods. Instead of synthesizing the presumed "active ingredients" from medicinal herbs, as done for prescription drugs, supplement manufacturers seek to extract and bottle the active ingredients from foods known or believed to promote good health and healing. And just like prescription drugs, the active agents function imperfectly, incompletely, and unpredictably when divorced from the whole-plant food from which they're derived or synthesized.[17]

Why would extracting nutrients from plants, or synthesizing them into supplements somehow be better for us than consuming the original foods in the way God (or nature) designed them? It doesn't make sense that the day-to-day health of human bodies would depend on the skills of modern food or health product manufacturers with their multimillion dollar processing plants and distribution systems. I'm not even sure some of the high-tech processing we do in our own kitchens lives up to the hype we hear. Our bodies evolved in low-tech environments through millions of years, and yet many people have become convinced that if we whip our food at 200 mph in an expensive Vitamix blender it will somehow be better for us.

I'm grateful we have many health options to choose from, but I am convinced we should begin our search for better health by choosing to follow the Word of Wisdom.

## Surely Individuals Differ in What Is Optimal for Them?

What about bodies that don't deal well with *all* wholesome plants? Whether through poor eating habits, unhealthy lifestyles, the environment, or genetics, some bodies do not presently deal well with certain whole foods. Some people are gluten intolerant.[18] Some get sick when they eat fruits that are perfectly fine for other people. Some don't like vegetables. Others don't do well on beans or certain grains. With all this variation, shouldn't we expect that different diets work best for different people? After all, it is a matter of fact that humans do survive on a wide variety of diets. Is there really a diet that is optimal for everyone, or do people vary too much from person to person?

While some people don't do well on certain plant foods, what is missing is evidence that animal, refined, or junk foods contribute to the optimal health of any individual. The fact that some people may "feel better" when they consume these products is no evidence of their healthful effects. There was a time when many Latter-day Saints felt their health required at least a little coffee, tea, alcohol or tobacco. After all, they didn't "feel good" when they did not consume these substances and using them made them "feel better." But what makes us feel good is not a wise standard for what will help us enjoy better health in the long run.

We all differ in various ways; this includes differences in cultures, family traditions, our environment and financial resources, as well as in our individual tastes. Nevertheless, while the Word of Wisdom does not dictate that particular plants *must* be eaten, it is clearly, in my opinion, not compatible with every dietary preference. There must be a reason the Word of Wisdom does not encourage us to just "eat right for your type."

Perhaps this is because the Word of Wisdom was primarily designed for one type—human beings.

Most animals have a particular diet that works well for them, and pet owners know what that diet is: cat owners do not feed their cats a diet of fruits and vegetables, nor do they feed chicken and fish to their rabbits.[19] A Word of Wisdom designed for lions, tigers, or bears would differ from that designed for humans. It is a blessing that humans are able to subsist on a wide variety of diets in times of necessity because at certain times our choices have been limited. Today, we rarely face these limitations; we have a great deal of choice and are blessed to know the type of diet that works best for human bodies so we can choose wisely.

While there is no doubt that certain people do not do well on certain plants, there are no particular plants mandated by the Word of Wisdom. Wheat is the only plant mentioned by name as being "for man." We are told that all wholesome plants are for our use, and since there is an endless variety of plant foods in the world, there is enough flexibility in the Word of Wisdom to allow for an extreme variety of food choices. Any number of people consuming a WFPB diet conforming to the Word of Wisdom could choose foods that differ quite remarkably from each other. The choices, variations, and combinations are literally infinite.

Before deciding our bodies need meat or processed foods that have no resemblance to wholesome plants, perhaps it would be worthwhile to try to find a diet that both works for us as individuals *and* meets the standard given by the Word of Wisdom.

## What about Moderation in All Things?

A low-fat whole food, plant-based diet is not a diet of "moderation in all things." It emphasizes eating whole, unrefined plant foods: vegetables, fruits, and grains (including legumes). Animal foods (meat, dairy, and eggs) are not recommended, except in times of genuine need. Oils, refined sugars, and other highly processed foods are not wholesome or prudent. While I think there are other legitimate interpretations of the counsel in the Word of Wisdom, this is the only diet that has been clinically proven to eliminate heart disease, and the same diet that is good for eliminating heart disease is good for eliminating other major chronic illness.[20] Therefore, I believe this diet gives us the best insight into how to interpret the Word of Wisdom and understand the optimal diet for human beings.

For many people, a low-fat WFPB diet seems radical. But which is more radical?

1. The SAD diet that is harmful to the human body and that guarantees most individuals will have a lower quality of life because they will suffer various chronic illnesses during their lifetimes?

or

2. The WFPB diet eaten by the vast majority of humans throughout recorded history that provides good nutrition and allows us to avoid most chronic illnesses?

As mentioned earlier, one out of every two men and one out of every three women in America will suffer from heart disease, a disease that is almost 100 percent preventable through eating this ostensibly radical diet. One in every three European-American children born in America today will develop diabetes during his or her lifetime. One out of every *two* Hispanic and African-American children face the same fate. Type 2 diabetes is, again, almost 100 percent preventable by eating the same radical diet. Add to that the many preventable strokes and cancers that members of our society will suffer. Why don't we consider the disease-inducing Standard American Diet the radical one?

I believe 50 years from now, we'll look back on this time and ask ourselves why we ever allowed our diet to evolve in such an unhealthy way to such disastrous results. We'll recognize then that our current SAD diet, in the context of history, was, without question, radical. As Dr. John McDougall puts it, "Open-heart surgery is radical. Eating oatmeal and potatoes is not radical."

What about moderation in all things? It makes sense to be moderate when all the choices are relatively good ones, but when some of the choices cause death and disease, it does not make sense to include these choices, even in moderate amounts. What if we smoked or drank or did drugs in moderate amounts? How well would that work? "Moderation in all things" is not a scriptural phrase, for good reason.

While it is true that if we only consumed small amounts of animal and junk foods (5 percent or less of our diet), chances are it would not have a significant impact on our health, the same is true of consuming small amounts of alcohol, tobacco, coffee or tea. If it were easy to keep all of these unhealthy foods to a minimum, we would not need the Word of Wisdom. Instead of aiming for "moderation," let's stick with "prudence" (D&C 89:11).

# Who Can Eat This Way?

The Word of Wisdom standard of eating wholesome plants "with prudence" (D&C 89:10–11) suggests a diet of primarily unrefined plant
foods. When I introduce people to this diet, they quickly realize it is very
different from the standard American diet. They are correct. On average,
Americans consume 51 percent refined and processed foods, 42 percent
dairy and animal foods, and a mere 7 percent fruits and vegetables.[21] A
WFPB diet excludes virtually *all* of the top ten sources of calories in the
American diet (as identified by the USDA): soda pop, cake and pastries,
hamburgers, pizza, potato chips, white rice, white bread, cheese, beer, and
french fries.[22]

Most people feel the effort required to make and sustain such a dramatic change in diet would be enormous. Some believe it is impossible.
Quite a few individuals (I used to be one of them!) can't imagine giving
up butter, cheese, or ice cream. Others won't sacrifice meat; still others,
processed foods, including vegetable oils and the oh-so-delicious variety
of high fat/high sugar treats of all kinds.

I admit that following this diet would mean a major change for most
people, and yet, despite our addiction to unhealthy foods and the very
powerful forces (think advertising, family, and friends) that help keep us
addicted, the Lord tells us that the Word of Wisdom is, "adapted to the
capacity of the weak and the weakest of all saints, who are or can be called
saints" (D&C 89:3). In other words, as difficult as the diet may appear at
first glance, the Lord knows better. He knows this diet is doable, even for
the "weakest."

As we know, most non-LDS people indulge in substances that are
forbidden in the Word of Wisdom: alcohol, tobacco, coffee and/or tea.
Ask them to give up their favorite habit, and they might quickly protest:
"That's impossible!" A great many people believe they cannot live without
their morning coffee or evening glass of wine. Even if we are fortunate
enough not to know what it is like to be addicted to such substances, we
understand giving them up can be extremely difficult. But is it impossible? Think of the hundreds of thousands of people who join the LDS
Church each year, most of whom do have to give up one or more of these
substances.

Last year during a Relief Society lesson in our ward on the Word of
Wisdom, one of the sisters, Diana Mahony, shared this personal experi-

ence, which illustrates that sacrifices are relative to what we feel we are getting in return:

> When I was young, we lived in Cleveland where the winters were cold and humid. We'd get chilled to the bone, so I started drinking coffee very early in life. The adults didn't see anything wrong with it. My grandmother added a little whiskey to my coffee so I wouldn't catch cold going to school. Later, she gave me warm milk with a little whiskey to treat cramps. By the time I was a teenager, I consumed coffee regularly every day. I was a diligent and ambitious student and felt coffee was needed to get me through studying late hours.
>
> But when I was 17, my junior year in high school, I went to an LDS cottage meeting that was missionary-oriented. They discussed the apostasy and the Restoration and Joseph Smith's First Vision and some converts bore their testimonies. I heard that, and I immediately said, "Yeah, that is true." It was so obvious to me. It rang like a bell. I never fasted, or studied, or prayed about it. I heard it and just felt, "Yeah, that is right." That is just the way it was.
>
> I went home and told my family I was going to join the Mormons, and they didn't think anything of it. They thought it was just a passing thing. But the next morning at breakfast, I passed up the coffee. I said, "Mormons don't drink coffee, so I'm not going to drink the coffee." I never drank coffee or alcohol again. I had no desire. The decision was made. I loved coffee, but I wanted to be a Mormon, and Mormons didn't drink coffee, so I didn't drink coffee. Period. That was it. I didn't have withdrawals. I was so excited about hearing the gospel, I could have given up breathing. It was like shedding a skin. Does a butterfly miss being a caterpillar?

When I talk with people about this diet, a few tell me they could never eat this way, that they don't have enough willpower. They admit this diet would be better for them, but they believe they are incapable of doing it. Because of D&C 89:3, I assume this is not true. Again, the diet is "adapted to the capacity of the *weak* and the *weakest* of all saints, who are or can be called saints." In truth, eating this way is much easier than living with heart disease, cancer, or paralysis from a stroke. How is it that people who feel they can't eat this way are nevertheless able to survive for *years* with chronic illness?

Compared to chronic illness, this diet is simple. It does involve learning a few new cooking skills and making some changes to our lifestyle, but it is not brain surgery or rocket science. It is simply switching to a diet of mostly whole, unrefined plant foods made into delicious meals and snacks. If this feels unnatural to us, it may be because we have grown up in a world of very unnatural foods.

Furthermore, a WFPB diet is not a diet of austerity. This earth was not created in such a way that Adam and Eve and their descendants did not have the pleasure of enjoying scrumptious foods until Chili's and the Cheesecake Factory opened for business. The Lord has blessed us with an earth filled with diverse plants of endless variety, taste, smell, and texture. I love these verses in D&C 59 that indicate God's delight in blessing us with the fullness of the earth:

> Yea, all things which come of the earth, in the season thereof, are made for the benefit and the use of man, both to please the eye and to gladden the heart; Yea, for food and for raiment, for taste and for smell, to strengthen the body and to enliven the soul. And it pleaseth God that he hath given all these things unto man. (D&C 59:18–20)

It is true that a child who grows up on Chicken McNuggets, french fries and soda pop will have a hard time adjusting to real food, but that is not because real food is not delicious. Even adults whose palates are accustomed to processed foods with layers of salt, fat, and sugar may need some time to acquire the ability to savor the more subtle delights of wholesome plant foods. Of course, it is easier for someone who grows up eating healthy food, but regardless of our age, we can do it.

Actually, most people I talk to don't say they *can't* do it; they frankly tell me they *don't want to do it.* And I understand that. Because the Church has not mandated it, we are (I think wisely) left to decide for ourselves the meaning of the Word of Wisdom and how we want to observe it. We get to choose for ourselves. The Church has spared us from the worst of problems by spelling out the things that are most harmful. But we get to choose how we pursue the promised blessings of "health in their navel and marrow to their bones . . . wisdom and great treasures of knowledge . . . run and not be weary, and . . . walk and not faint" (D&C 89:18–20).

For me, the choice was not hard. When I consider the precious promises in the Word of Wisdom, the sacrifices seem very small compared with these blessings. I want to be the butterfly!

# Real Mormons ✤ Real Stories

## *Mavis's Story*

My parents were very health conscious. We ate only "healthy" *raw* sugar; white sugar was never allowed in the house. Breakfast consisted of hot cereal, covered with liberal amounts of *unpasteurized* cream from the registered Brown Swiss dairy cows my brother raised. We used only whole-wheat bread on our daily lunch of grilled-cheese sandwiches (smothered in large quantities of margarine). We always had a salad and a "proper" two servings of vegetables with our meat every night for dinner (though I never bothered to actually *eat* the salad *or* the vegetables . . . ), and we always had a glass of fresh, unpasteurized milk with every meal, and lots of pure ice cream for dessert. Of course, I now know that most everything we *thought* was healthy turned out to be otherwise, but back then we were proud of our careful diet . . .

Growing up in a "proper" LDS home, I learned very young that the Word of Wisdom—no alcohol, coffee, tea, or tobacco—was an important part of our religion. I never actually *read* Section 89, but I fervently believed in it. Of course, by *not* bothering to read the Lord's counsel, I was easily deceived by every fad I was exposed to—and there were many—*all* to which I fell prey.

I learned from the Starch Blocker pills that were so popular when I was in high school that "starch" was something "bad." How exciting that someone came up with a way to allow me to eat all the pizza and pasta I wanted! Too bad it didn't work . . .

When the Atkins Diet came out, I joyfully ate huge quantities of eggs, bacon, butter, steak, hamburger, sausage, pork rinds, and cheese—and kept a lithe figure—as long as I ate only those foods . . . But I found myself dreaming about apples and tomatoes and potatoes and peas—all those nasty high-carbohydrate items I wasn't allowed—and I found myself going on binges of the starchy "no-no's"—and, of course, gaining weight.

My husband, a devoted and loving doctor, put me on every new diet he read about in his medical journals: First, Medifast, where I got a delicious (highly processed) 150-calorie chocolate shake four times a day—which worked great—until I couldn't stand starving any longer.

Then along came the marvelous appetite suppressant Fen-Phen, which I took for years—until I found out one day that yes, I, too, like thousands of other women taking it, had heart damage.

I, of course, used liberal amounts of the wonderful "heart-healthy" olive oil and exotic, pure-plant coconut oil (so useful for cooking with high heat), and coconut cream added so much flavor to everything I cooked. And, like everyone else, I indulged in the latest craze—*fat-free Greek* yogurt—which I religiously ate by the quart (with strawberries) every morning for breakfast—as I kept gaining weight . . .

At last I found the ultimate "cure" for obesity: hCG. Just two drops under my tongue twice a day (and a very strict diet) enabled me to lose 50 pounds! But as soon as I went off hCG, the weight started coming back again. So I did another regimen of hCG—only it didn't work very well the second time around . . . So I tried it *again*, and the *third* time, it didn't work at all . . .

In desperation, I prayed fervently for help to keep from gaining all the weight back. That very week I was assigned a new visiting teacher: Jane Birch. Although she had no idea of my struggle with weight, she suggested that I might be interested in the DVD *Forks Over Knives*. By the end of that DVD, I was a believer in a whole food, plant-based diet—and I have never looked back. I have found that a WFPB diet is delicious, satisfying, and filling. Having always been a *quantity* eater, I can enjoy eating large servings of salads and vegetables to my heart's content, without needing to (in fact I *refuse to)* count calories any more. I now have an appreciation and understanding of the wisdom the Lord gave us so many years ago *that I never bothered to really read.*

*Mavis Parkinson is from Provo, Utah and has a Master of Arts Degree in Theater History from BYU. She taught theatre in high schools and universities and is currently on the board of the Utah Shakespeare Festival. However, her first love is spending time with family and grandchildren!*

# 8

# Stewards of Our Bodies, the Earth, and Its Creatures

Central to understanding the Word of Wisdom is an understanding of the absolutely critical role of the body in both our mortal experience and in the eternities. I am not sure any of us fully comprehend the importance of having a physical body, or understand how sacred our bodies are. The Apostle Paul taught:

> . . . Know ye not that your body is the temple of the Holy Ghost which is in you, which ye have of God, and ye are not your own? For ye are bought with a price: therefore glorify God in your body, and in your spirit, which are God's. (1 Cor. 6:19–20)

We are the literal children of God. Our bodies are made in His image. They are gifts from our Father, and we are stewards over them, to keep and protect them. We do not want to pollute our bodies any more than our spirits, for they are "the temple of the Holy Ghost." Just think what an endowment we were given when we came to this mortal world and entered these tabernacles of God (D&C 93:35).

We are likewise stewards over this beautiful earth, to keep and protect it as a sacred and precious gift. After creating this earth and all the creatures thereon, God proclaimed them to be good. God loves not just us, but the whole earth, and all the creatures on it. In fact, God gave commandments not just to us, but also to all His creatures. And He covenanted not just with us, but also with every living creature (Genesis 9:8–15).

We are not told in detail all the covenants the creatures of this earth made. We know that they, like us, were commanded to multiply and replenish the earth (Genesis 1:22). But we also know animals have a role to play in the preservation of human life:

> And whoso forbiddeth to abstain from meats, that man should not eat the same, is not ordained of God;
>
> For, behold, the beasts of the field and the fowls of the air, and that which cometh of the earth, is *ordained for the use of man* for food and for raiment, and that he might have *in abundance*. (D&C 49:18–19, emphasis added; see note for expanded analysis of this verse in relationship to 1 Timothy 4:3[1])

I am humbled by these verses and the understanding that God's amazing animal creatures have been ordained for our use. However, just as God ordained these creatures for our use, He makes it plain what the boundaries of that use are. Continuing from the above verses we read:

> But it is not given that one man should possess that which is *above another*, wherefore the world lieth in sin.
>
> And *wo be unto man that sheddeth blood or that wasteth flesh and hath no need.* (D&C 49:20–21, emphasis added)

The same principle is taught in D&C 59:

> Verily I say, that inasmuch as ye do this, the fulness of the earth is yours, the beasts of the field and the fowls of the air, and that which climbeth upon the trees and walketh upon the earth;
>
> . . . Yea, for food and for raiment, for taste and for smell, to strengthen the body and to enliven the soul.
>
> And it pleaseth God that he hath given all these things unto man; for unto this end were they made to be used, *with judgment, not to excess, neither by extortion.* (D&C 59:16, 19–20, emphasis added)

God has given us rich abundance, but He also has commanded us to be wise stewards. He has ordained the use of animals to sustain our lives in times of need, but we are told to use judgment and to not shed blood when there is no need. Furthermore, this injunction is not just a modern commandment. In the beginning, God gave our first parents a diet of plants. In the Bible account, consuming the flesh of animals is introduced only after the flood destroyed the vegetation on the earth. In Joseph Smith's translation of Genesis, we learn that God tells Noah that now he may eat meat, but He emphasizes its use only in times of need:

> Every moving thing that liveth shall be meat for you; even as
> the green herb have I given you all things. . . .
>
> And surely, blood shall not be shed, only for meat, to save
> your lives; and the blood of every beast will I require at your
> hands. (JST Genesis 9:9, 11)

I have been emphasizing the health reasons why we should be careful
about our meat consumption, but it is perhaps our duty to be good stewards of the earth and of the animals that is equally pleasing to the Lord.

I do not doubt that one role of animals is to serve as food for humans.
We are told several times that they are ordained for our *use*, but that does
not mean they are ordained for our *abuse*.[2] The Lord gave humans dominion over the animals, just as He gives parents dominion over their children.[3] We are blessed with this opportunity, and we are privileged to act
in the place of God to serve those weaker than ourselves. This is a sacred
stewardship for which we will be held accountable.

God has blessed us with rich abundance, and this is pleasing to Him.
But He asks us to use these blessings with judgment, to use the flesh of
animals "sparingly," only in times of need. Hugh Nibley suggests the use
of the word *sparing* means "sparing God's creatures." Nibley goes on to say,

> The family who needs a deer to get through the winter have
> a right to that. The Lord will not deny them, but He is also
> pleased with those who forbear.[4]
>
> God will justify the taking of animal life to sustain man's
> want, but he reserves a special blessing for those who place
> their own nobility before their necessity.[5]

I can imagine a possible scene from long ago: God asking the animals
if they would be willing to perform the sacrifice of giving their lives for
humans when the need arose. I imagine them agreeing to do this for us,
perhaps even knowing that at times we'd abuse that privilege. This, of
course, is speculation on my part, but it nevertheless strengthens the love
and respect I feel for these fellow creatures who in so many ways enrich
our common world, and who are often called on to sacrifice their lives
for our sakes. Why should we take advantage of their relative weakness?

## Plant Foods are Better for the Earth and the Animals

Only after I stopped consuming animal flesh did I become aware of
how abusive mankind can be in how we treat animals to obtain, not

just food for times of need, but food in excess, food for pleasure, food for game, food that we indulge in because we can afford to do so, and far more food than most of our brothers and sisters in foreign lands can ever hope to obtain.

I will not go into detail here elaborating the problems with the meat, dairy, and egg industries, but the treatment of animals in these food factories is surely antithetical to the verses I've just quoted from the D&C, in which we are asked to use animals "with judgment, not to excess, neither by extortion" (D&C 59:20). Animals are routinely held in what can only be described as abusive conditions, where they are caged in small areas, allowed no freedom, are continually administered drugs to keep them alive, and are fattened quickly for the slaughter.[6] They are not allowed to freely fulfill God's commandment to multiply and replenish the earth, nor are they allowed to fulfill their natural biological instincts to care for their young. Humans take this entire process into their own hands so they can manipulate these lives for their own profit. Under these conditions, how could these animals take joy in fulfilling the measure of their creation? The animal food industry works hard to make sure we do not witness the conditions in which animals are kept in order to produce the amount of animal foods eaten in this country. They are well aware that most people, when exposed to the facts, would be morally outraged.[7]

Likewise, I've learned that the production of meat and dairy products has an inordinate impact on the environment. It is not widely understood how much more energy, land, water, and other resources are required to produce animal foods versus plant foods.[8] In California, for example, it takes roughly 25 gallons of water to produce a pound of lettuce, tomatoes, potatoes or wheat; 49 gallons for apples; 815 gallons for chicken; 1,630 gallons for pork; and a whopping 5,214 gallons of water for a pound of beef. You would save more water by not eating one pound of California beef than you would by not showering for six months.[9]

Raising animals for food is a highly inefficient use of resources; we must devote an enormous quantity of food (the *majority* of the grain and cereals we grow in this country) to feed animals to produce a comparatively small amount of meat, dairy, and eggs. We could instead directly consume the food we feed the animals with much less cost to the environment and to our health (not to mention the health of the animals!). Not only could we feed ourselves, we'd have enough food left over to feed all of the world's poor.[10] I like the fact that by reducing our animal food consumption and devoting those resources to feeding the poor, we could not only dramatically improve our health, but also bless our brothers and sisters around the world. This seems right in light of the following scripture:

> But it is not given that one man should possess that which is above another, wherefore the world lieth in sin. And wo be unto man that sheddeth blood or that wasteth flesh and hath no need. (D&C 49:20–21)

Furthermore, we all know how vulnerable we are due to the volatile supply of readily available fossil fuels. We are also increasingly aware of the environmental impact of how we use these fuels, which disproportionally affects the poor of the world.[11] We use an enormous amount of energy to fuel our cars, trucks, airplanes, buses, and motorcycles, and the chemical gases they emit may be wreaking havoc on the environment worldwide. Yet, livestock production produces more greenhouse gases than all forms of transportation combined.[12] While I struggle to imagine our modern world functioning without modern transportation, what would we lose by giving up meat, dairy, and eggs? (Hint: heart disease, strokes, diabetes, pollution, etc.)

According to a careful study done at the University of Chicago, people who consume animal foods are responsible for an extra ton and a half of $CO_2$ equivalent per person per year, as compared to people who consume no animal foods.[13] As a consequence, a person who changes from an animal-based diet to a plant-based diet would save more greenhouse emissions per year than switching from a Toyota Camry to a hybrid Toyota Prius (at much less cost!). If everyone on the planet switched to a low-meat diet, such a transition would dramatically impact our ability to resolve environmental issues that now appear intractable. One estimate suggests such a global change "would reduce the mitigation costs to achieve a 450 ppm $CO_2$ -eq. stabilization target by about 50 percent in 2050."[14]

In a study comparing vegetarian and non-vegetarian diets, "the non-vegetarian diet required 2.9 times more water, 2.5 times more primary energy, 13 times more fertilizer, and 1.4 times more pesticides than did the vegetarian diet."[15] The livestock industry is "by far the single largest anthropogenic user of land," a leading contributor to deforestation and land degradation, and a major factor in the reduction of biodiversity.[16] And livestock produce 130 times more waste in the US than humans do, leading to widespread pollution of land and water.[17] Unfortunately, these are just a few of the disconcerting facts that can be cited about the environmental costs of animal food production. Bill McKibben, a well-respected voice for the environment, concludes, "Industrial livestock production is essentially indefensible—ethically, ecologically, and otherwise."[18]

We in America seem to feel it is our right to eat whatever amount of animal foods we can afford, but this practice is not sustainable in the long run, especially as the world's population grows and demands the same right. As Philip Wollen (former VP of Citibank) stated in a passionate address in defense of animals, "The earth can produce enough for everyone's *need*, but not enough for everyone's *greed*."[19] The Lord tells us He has blessed us with rich abundance, that "the earth is full, and there is enough and to spare" (D&C 104:17). Only our greed makes it otherwise. A WFPB diet is not just healthy and humane; it is also sustainable. It helps us fulfill our responsibility as wise stewards of this beautiful world.

Since changing my diet, my love and appreciation for this planet has deepened significantly. Just as we depend on this earth, the earth depends on us. We are intimately interrelated, and I'm concerned that she groans under our sins. The biological and physical worlds are pure. They fully obey the will of the Lord and are redeemed through their service to us, but they also suffer due to our disobedience. I believe we humans are the cause of much of the "natural" chaos in the world. It is a reflection of who we are and of the choices we have made. Brigham Young said:

> Let the people be holy, and the earth under their feet will be holy. Let the people be holy, and filled with the Spirit of God, and every animal and creeping thing will be filled with peace; the soil of the earth will bring forth in its strength, and the fruits thereof will be meat for man. The more purity that exists, the less is the strife; the more kind we are to our animals, the more will peace increase, and the savage nature of the brute creation vanish away.[20]

I believe that ceasing enmity toward animals will lead to a greater depth of spirituality, sensitivity, and charity in the hearts of the Latter-day Saints and help prepare the earth for the Millennium. We must change for harmony to exist in the world of nature and things. Only then can we be fully at peace with each other and with all of God's creatures.

# Encouragement from LDS Leaders

Beginning with Joseph Smith, latter-day prophets and other LDS Church leaders have spoken out frequently and with great eloquence on the responsibility we humans have for our fellow creatures.[21] For example, Joseph Smith related the following experience from the 1834 Zion's Camp expedition:

> In pitching my tent we found three massasaugas or prairie rattlesnakes, which the brethren were about to kill, but I said, "Let them alone—don't hurt them! How will the serpent ever lose his venom, while the servants of God possess the same disposition, and continue to make war upon it? Men must become harmless, before the brute creation; and when men lose their vicious dispositions and cease to destroy the animal race, the lion and the lamb can dwell together, and the sucking child can play with the serpent in safety." The brethren took the serpents carefully on sticks and carried them across the creek. I exhorted the brethren not to kill a serpent, bird, or an animal of any kind during our journey unless it became necessary in order to preserve ourselves from hunger.[22]

Apostle George Q. Cannon wrote:

> [God] has bestowed life upon man, and upon beasts, birds, fishes and insects, and no one has the right to take that life, except in the way and under the conditions which the Lord prescribes.
>
> . . . when man becomes their true friend, [the animals] will learn to love and not to fear him. The Spirit of the Lord which will rest upon man will also be given to the animal creation—man will not hurt nor destroy, not even tigers and lions and wolves and snakes, and they will not harm him— and universal peace will prevail.[23]

One reason Church leaders may have felt so strongly about this issue is that the Latter-day Saint view on animals is fairly unique among Christians. We believe animals, like humans, are eternal beings (see D&C 77:2–3); that they are "living souls" (Moses 3:19) who will be "resurrected and glorified" in God's presence;[24] and that we are accountable to God for our stewardship over them (see JST Genesis 9:5 and D&C 104:11–14). Regarding animals, Heber C. Kimball wrote, "Let them rest: They are as good as we are in their sphere of action; they honour their calling, and we do not, when we abuse them: they have the same life in them that you have, and we should not hurt them."[25]

Other Church leaders have spoken out with care and passion for animals and emphasized our responsibility to not hurt or kill them, except as needed for food. Apostle Lorenzo Snow said, "We have no right to slay animals or fowls except from necessity, for they have spirits which may someday rise up and accuse or condemn us."[26] Apostle Joseph Fielding Smith further explained, "Although there was no sin in the shedding of their blood when required for food . . . to take the life of these creatures wantonly is a sin before the Lord. It is easy to destroy life, but who can restore it when it is taken?"[27]

President Joseph F. Smith, in particular, was well known for his kindness to animals. He spoke and wrote often about our obligation toward them. The year he died, he made a profound statement that was "later quoted by two other prophets":[28]

> We are a part of all life and should study carefully our relationship to it. We should be in sympathy with it, and not allow our prejudices to create a desire for its destruction. The unnecessary destruction of life begets a spirit of destruction which grows within the soul. It lives by what it feeds upon and robs man of the love that he should have for the works of God. . . . The unnecessary destruction of life is a distinct spiritual loss to the human family. Men can not worship the Creator and look with careless indifference upon his creations. The love of all life helps man to the enjoyment of a better life. . . . Wisdom and virtue come from the animal and vegetable world which carries with it a spiritual as well as a material blessing. Nature helps us to see and understand God. To all His creations we owe an allegiance of service and a profound admiration. . . . Love of nature is akin to the love of God, the two are inseparable.[29]

I am impressed that the same diet that is optimal for the human body is also good to the earth and kind to the animals. Surely this, too, is more in keeping with the Word of Wisdom.

# Real Mormons ❧ Real Stories

## *Doug's Story*

When I read the Word of Wisdom, there is a phrase that really touches me. Speaking of the animals, the Lord says, "it is pleasing unto me that they should not be used" (D&C 89:13). It is pleasing to Him. What a choice emotion for the Lord to say He has. It sounds like a very good thing to me.

I have never seen an animal die in person. I've definitely seen them alive though. And they are so alive. They enjoy the company of their kind. They see and experience things. There is something good and innocent in all of them. At this point, if I needed to eat one, I'd like it to be for a special reason, not just because it tastes good, but because I need some food for my family to eat and there is nothing else. In that case, I would gratefully use them as food.

Perhaps part of God's way of showing us His gladness is naturally rewarding us with better health when we eat closer to what He would prefer. From the many reputable scientific studies I have read, food we create based on animal flesh, eggs, or milk seems to cause harm. Animal foods lead toward debilitating disease at worst and are an organ-burdening fuel at best. None of the supposed benefits outweigh the long-term harm.

So I see animals differently now, which I only let myself do once they weren't food anymore. I like thinking about all of their big and little lives, full of their own emotions and struggles, being left alone to live in their way. I think I understand a little of what is pleasing to our Savior, who is full of understanding of all creatures, knows their enjoyment and pain as intimately as ours, and whose bowels are full of mercy for all He has suffered. That may sound silly to some people, but I think it is far from it.

There were a lot of questions I had when my wife and I started considering eating this way. There were concerns about adequate nutrition, enough protein, and whether humans could be healthy without calcium from milk. With reassurance from the Word of Wisdom, I went to work studying the scientific literature. I soon discovered how misguided those concerns were.

Although I was healthy when I started this diet, I was surprised to receive added health benefits. For example, after I switched to a whole food, plant-based diet, I rather casually beat my high school personal best mile time on a track, without training for it. Later, I took first place in my age division at the Rex Lee 5k Run. I attribute this and improved eyesight to better blood flow and muscle efficiency without so much fat in the blood.

I stopped eating meat, eggs, and dairy for selfish reasons. I wouldn't call myself a vegan. Ethical vegans can live on fries and Oreos if their main concern is the animals. They're not necessarily doing it to be healthy. But I now understand ethical vegans, instead of pitying them. Their reasons have an overabundance of merit. The ominous environmental reasons are also enough on their own to warrant eating grains and other starches instead of animal products. It just turns out that the best thing for a human is the best thing for the planet, including water conservation and the economy. Not to mention the animals themselves, who I'm sure would prefer to not live in often lightless, cramped, filthy conditions nor constantly drink water laced with antibiotics just to survive and grow quickly in that harsh environment (unnervingly causing the rapid evolution of antibiotic-resistant superbugs in these factories). Such factories will continue to be necessary if humans continue to eat them at the same rate we do now.

This message can be difficult to share with others, including Mormons. Copious amounts of ice cream seem justifiable in a culture that has eliminated more standard vices like alcohol. I understand that we're all sensitive and protective of how we feel about ourselves and how others view us. I feel that it is important to let each individual know that, in my view, they are fantastic. I admire them. They are better than me in countless ways. There are things I should be asking them about their knowledge and experience that I'm still ignorant of. Only with this attitude and understanding can anything meaningful be shared from my end. Love, respect, and honor matter deeply to all of us.

The Word of Wisdom rings true to my mind, and especially to my heart. As I learn of the abuse billions of farmed animals go through daily, I can't help hearing the Lord's "it is pleasing unto me that they should not be used" as a loving request on behalf of many innocent beings. God has provided a better way, one brimming with love, abundance, and real health for us, for the earth, and for the other beings we share it with.

*Doug Hawkes is 29 years old and studies bioinformatics at BYU in Provo, Utah. In the summer you might find him at a Kiwanis Park pickup soccer game. Join in and judge his claim that he can still play faster than the guys fresh out of high school. He and his wife Stephanie love getting lost together hiking in the mountains whenever they can.*

# 9

# Why Doesn't the Church Tell Us These Things?

I think it is interesting that in Joseph Smith's inspired introduction to the Word of Wisdom, he stated this scripture was given

> . . . *not by commandment or constraint*, but by revelation and the word of wisdom, showing forth the order and will of God in the *temporal* salvation of all saints in the last days. (D&C 89:2–3, emphasis added)

The word *temporal* seems important. Why temporal? Why not *eternal* salvation? Could it be that keeping every aspect of the Word of Wisdom is not requisite for our eternal salvation but is rather a blessing for our temporal well-being in this life? Elder Heber J. Grant observed in 1895:

> I want to say that some of the sweetest spirited men whom I have ever known, and men as true to the Gospel as I ever could be, have disobeyed the Word of Wisdom.[1]

Elder Grant was referring to the prohibitions of the Word of Wisdom, but the same could be said about the rest of the counsel in Section 89. As far as I know, none of our modern-day prophets have eaten a strict vegetarian diet, but surely they, and many other meat-eating Saints we know, are among the most spiritual people to have walked this earth. But were they the healthiest? Could even a saint enjoy better health by more fully keeping the Word of Wisdom?

## A Look Back at Church History

From the beginning, many Church leaders and members accepted the Word of Wisdom as a commandment from God and felt strongly about the importance of keeping it. Some were even over-zealous in their desire to enforce it.[2] But for many Saints, learning to live the Word of Wisdom was a challenge. I suspect God knew that meeting this challenge would involve a very long process. And in fact, it took about 100 years before strict obedience to the Church policy on the Word of Wisdom came to be widely accepted as the standard expected of all faithful Church members.[3]

When the Word of Wisdom was revealed, alcohol, tobacco, coffee, and tea were widely used both inside and outside of the Church. While many contemporary advocates for better health practices condemned the use of these stimulants (along with many other foods, drinks, and practices they found unwholesome), their advocacy was not based on modern scientific evidence, as the professional study of nutrition was in its infancy. Furthermore, others championed the *benefits* of alcohol, tobacco, coffee, and tea for fatigue or special medical needs, and they were used widely to treat all kinds of illnesses (often in ways we'd find appalling today). In fact, the use of these stimulants for health was so common it seems to have not occurred to the early Saints that the Word of Wisdom should apply to those circumstances. Given the dominant cultural practices of the day and the wording "not by commandment or constraint" included in the revelation's introduction, many Saints interpreted it to warn only against serious abuse, drunkenness, and overindulgence.

While some early Saints were serious about applying a stricter interpretation to the Word of Wisdom, the majority, including many leaders, were much more liberal. The Prophet Joseph himself stressed forgiveness and charity over strict enforcement, and his immediate successors followed suit. After all, there were many more pressing issues during the decades following the revelation, like aiding the Saints in fleeing from persecutions, crossing the plains, settling the West, and keeping the economy from collapsing.

From the Nauvoo period to the 1880s, strict observance of the Word of Wisdom was largely an individual choice. Rather than stressing complete abstinence from all alcohol, tobacco, coffee, and tea, nineteenth-century Church leaders took more pragmatic positions, which included moderation, exceptions, and tolerance. President Brigham Young did not himself fully commit to the Word of Wisdom until the 1860s. As Church leaders began to fully commit, they were in a much better position to help lay members, but even then they were comparatively tolerant (especially toward older Saints), and even occasionally backtracked on encouraging strict obedience to the Word of Wisdom for various reasons, including economic ones.[4]

To me it is important to realize that even during times when the prohibitions listed in the Word of Wisdom were not mandated for faithful Latter-day Saints, those who followed these teachings were still blessed, not just spiritually, but also with better health. Even today non-members of the Church are blessed if they abstain from alcohol, tobacco, coffee, and tea, so it is clear that *it does not take a mandate from Church leaders to gain blessings from following counsel given in the Word of Wisdom.*

Helping Church members take the Word of Wisdom seriously and transition to the point where we are today was a long and arduous journey. It took decades of hard work and continual preaching. Church leaders were often discouraged by the enormous effort and continued reluctance of many Saints to obey. They did have help and support from some members. One prominent LDS woman wrote the following in 1877:

> Do we as a people realize the importance of those precious words. . . . Could we find fifty Latter-day Saints in the Territory who abstain from tea, coffee, whiskey and tobacco or considers that it is worth while to even give it a thought. Is it not high time to wake up and open our eyes and look about us. If the Lord had no purpose in giving the Word of Wisdom, why did he take the trouble to give it. And if it is not necessary for us to observe it, what is the use of having it.[5]

But while some Saints felt strongly about living the Word of Wisdom, others were largely oblivious. Even at the turn of the century, almost 70 years after the revelation, some Saints did not fully understand that their religion asked them to forego *all* alcohol, tobacco, coffee, and tea. After all, it was possible that their fellow ward members, even their bishops and stake presidents, might not have been fully keeping the Word of Wisdom. Members of the Church at that time could have smoked their way to lung cancer or drunk their way to cirrhosis of the liver, and still not have made a connection between their suffering and a lack of keeping the Word of Wisdom. (Fast forward to today: how many Saints see no connection between their heart disease or diabetes and their disregard for the advice given in D&C 89?)

President Heber J. Grant is well remembered as an ardent champion of the Word of Wisdom. He loved the Word of Wisdom and spoke on it often, even though he frequently felt his words were falling on deaf ears. You can feel his exasperation as he relates the following stories, which he shared during the 1895 General Conference as a young apostle:

> I confess to you ... that I have been humiliated beyond expression to go to one of the Stakes of Zion, to stand up and preach to the people and call upon them to obey the Word of Wisdom, and then to sit down to the table of a President of a Stake, after having preached with all the zeal, energy, and power that I possessed, calling upon the people to keep the commandments of God, and to have his wife ask me if I would like a cup of tea or a cup of coffee. I have felt in my heart that it was an insult, considering the words that I had spoken, and I have felt humiliated to think that I had not sufficient power, and enough of the Spirit of God to enable me to utter words that would penetrate the heart of a President of a Stake, that he at least would be willing to carry out the advice which I had given. I remember going to a Stake of Zion but a short time ago and preaching with all the energy I possessed and with all the Spirit that God would give me upon the necessity of refraining from the drinking of tea and coffee, and I heard also at that conference a very eloquent appeal to the Latter-day Saints by a man who, I understood, was a president of a quorum of Seventy. But when we came to take our meal, he jokingly said that he could not do without his tea and coffee, and he proposed to have it and suffer the consequences. I remember going to another Stake of Zion and preaching to the people on the necessity of refraining from tea and coffee and giving some figures upon the wasting of the people's means; and the president of the Stake remarked, after I got through, that he thought the Lord would forgive them if they did drink their coffee, because the water in that Stake of Zion was very bad. I did not say anything, but I thought a good deal, and I had to pray to the Lord and to bite my tongue....I have become so discouraged, so disheartened, so humiliated in my feelings.[6]

In the same speech, Elder Grant goes on to describe how discouraging it was that the Saints were spending more money breaking the Word of Wisdom than they were spending to keep the law of tithing! Despite his discouragement, Elder Grant continued to preach on the Word of Wisdom, even to the point of wearying many Saints. In 1932, as president of the Church, he stated that "he had been called a crank for constantly urging the Saints to observe the Word of Wisdom, but mentioned that he expected to be a crank in that respect to the end of his life."[7]

Notwithstanding the struggles, over the many decades definite progress was made, and more and more Saints became compliant with the Word of Wisdom. Finally, during President Grant's term as president of the Church, the time had arrived to enforce strict abstinence from alcohol, tobacco, coffee and tea as a requirement for a temple recommend and other Church privileges. During President Grant's tenure, abstaining from all alcohol, tobacco, coffee, and tea "came to be regarded as a binding principle [and] a test of individual obedience and worthiness."[8] Again, this was roughly 100 years after the revelation had first been given!

We owe a lot to these early leaders and Church members who, to their credit, did not give up in the face of a very difficult challenge. They not only changed their own behavior, they worked diligently to help their fellow Saints do the same. But it took much more than a revelation from God to bring this change to pass. Perhaps we shouldn't be surprised if the word of the Lord is not enough to persuade most Saints to pay attention to the rest of the counsel in Section 89.

## Why the Preoccupation with the Prohibitions?

Why have the D&C 89 prohibitions against using certain substances been stressed over the admonitions for consuming what is healthy? One obvious reason may be because the prohibitions very clearly contradicted the early Saints' dietary practices and forced them to reconsider the use of substances they regularly enjoyed. On the other hand, there would be no reason for them to focus on the advice regarding plants, grains, and meat, as their dietary practices did not obviously contradict that counsel. Subsequent Church leaders may have been more likely to focus on the prohibitions for the same reasons, and also because it is much easier to judge compliance if the commandment is specific.[9] In time, it also became clear that the consequences of disobeying the prohibitions, at least in terms of alcohol and tobacco, were critical for obvious health and social reasons.

In addition, if the time and effort that went into getting the Saints to obey the prohibitions of the Word of Wisdom is any example, perhaps another reason Church leaders have not encouraged strict observance to all the counsel in Section 89 is that Church members have not been ready to fully embrace it. Early Church leaders taught that they could not fully reveal to the people all that the Lord revealed to them because the people would not accept it. In 1844, just a few months before he was martyred, Joseph Smith said:

> I have tried for a number of years to get the minds of the Saints prepared to receive the things of God; but we frequently see some of them, after suffering all they have for the work of God, will fly to pieces like glass as soon as anything comes that is contrary to their traditions: they cannot stand the fire at all.[10]

Sometimes in conversations with others about the Word of Wisdom, I sense people are afraid to even open the door to the possibility that the Lord might prompt them to change how they eat. I certainly do not feel that everyone who studies the Word of Wisdom will be prompted to eat like I do, but I find it interesting that we sometimes fear even opening the door to these revelations. I am sure I only recognize this fear because I've experienced it many times in the past about any number of topics. We don't always welcome revelation. Elder George A. Smith commented on this phenomenon in 1855:

> . . . we find plainly illustrated, in the whole history contained in the sacred book, the principle that the Lord wished to reveal unto the children of men things which had been hid from before the foundation of the world, principles which would exalt them to celestial thrones, but they would not, or, which amounts to the same, He could never find a people, could never communicate with a generation or a very numerous body of men that would obey His commandments, listen to His counsel, and observe His wisdom, or be led by His revelations.[11]

Elder Smith describes occasions when the Lord could not "reveal to us a single principle farther than He had done" or "He would have upset the whole of us." Due to unbelief, the Lord had to very carefully reveal His will:

> [He had to] be so careful, and advance the idea so slowly, to communicate them to the children of men with such great caution that, at all hazards, a few of them might be able to understand and obey.[12]

We are told the Lord will bless us with "commandments not a few" (D&C 59:4). What would our lives be like if we loved and embraced *all* the commandments the Lord blesses us with? Of course, the Word of Wisdom is not the only revelation we do not fully keep. Who among us is totally honest, has complete faith, always serves unselfishly, and thinks kind thoughts about drivers who rudely cut us off? We know the Lord's blessings are not reserved for only those who are perfect, and that He will bless us to the full extent He is able as we learn "line upon line, precept upon precept" (2 Nephi 28:30). I believe we Latter-day Saints truly want to do what is right, but our lives are already very complicated, and considering a change in diet can be overwhelming. If I can understand this, I know God certainly understands this.

Finally, like many religious peoples, we tend to focus our attention on prohibitions (the "thou shalt nots") even when we realize that the admonitions are equally, indeed often more, important (e.g., love neighbor, keep the Sabbath day holy, forget ourselves in service). Perhaps not doing the wrong is a stepping-stone to doing the right. Perhaps learning to obey the Word of Wisdom prohibitions has been a stepping-stone for the Latter-day Saints. Now that we pretty much have that step down, are we ready for the next step?

## We are Not Very Different from the Early Saints!

I find the history of the Word of Wisdom very interesting in light of my evolving understanding of this revelation. There are many interesting parallels between (1) how the early Saints viewed the Word of Wisdom prohibitions, and (2) the views of Saints today toward the so-called "positive aspects" of the Word of Wisdom:

- We take a liberal view of the parts of the Word of Wisdom not specifically mandated or enforced by Church leaders, and most of us, including Church leaders, do not strictly follow the non-mandated admonitions.
- We interpret the Word of Wisdom based on our knowledge of science, the customs of the wider culture, and the traditions we've grown up with.
- We are so prejudiced by our current understanding of sound health practices that we discount parts of the Word of Wisdom

that go against it, or we reinterpret those verses to fit our understanding.

- We can't believe using certain substances can be all that bad
  when we observe that most good Latter-day Saints, including
  most Church leaders, are consuming them.

- We are reluctant to change unless someone in authority spells
  it out for us, and (equally importantly) we see everyone around
  us doing it. (As President Grant discovered, it takes more than
  direct admonition to get most of us to change our behavior!)

- Social customs and our intense desire to be a gracious host or
  guest have a powerful effect on our actions, even to the point
  of contradicting what we know to be good advice (think of the
  stake president's wife offering President Grant tea and coffee).

- We feel justified in ignoring advice in the Word of Wisdom
  when it doesn't suit our health needs and bodily constitution:
  I need meat; I can't eat grains; I don't like vegetables, etc. (As
  mentioned earlier, many early Saints excused their use of coffee,
  tea, liquor, and/or tobacco because they felt their body did not
  function well without these substances.)

- Our natural inclination is to emphasize "moderation."

- Once we are accustomed to using substances not good for our
  bodies, it is very difficult for us to change the way we eat.

- We (very rightly) feel other aspects of the gospel (e.g., charity,
  service) are more important than "fanatical" observance of the
  Word of Wisdom.

- We believe (again, rightly) that there are many issues the Church
  faces that are far more important than how we eat. For today's
  Church, this may include issues like pornography, sexual abuse,
  and the breakdown of families.

Vegetarianism is obviously not a Mormon doctrine. We do not believe
humans should never consume meat under any circumstance. Church
leaders do not preach veganism from the pulpit. It is not a question asked
in temple recommend interviews. Animal foods are served routinely (and
not even sparingly) in the Church Office Building, Brigham Young University, and other Church-operated facilities.

On the other hand, mandatory meat consumption is also not part of
our religion. *There is absolutely no prohibition against Latter-day Saints*

*adopting a plant-based diet or enthusiastically encouraging others to do so*, though of course it is not our prerogative to command others to abstain from meats.[13]

Like the early Saints, though neither Church leaders nor members are necessarily leading the way, it does not stop us from gaining blessings, both spiritual and temporal, by voluntarily choosing to more closely follow the Lord's advice. In admonishing the early Saints to obey the Word of Wisdom, President Grant reminds us, "it is not meet that we should be commanded in all things."[14]

The early Saints, as a whole, did not manage to fully abstain from the substances prohibited in the Word of Wisdom until Church leaders more or less commanded it by making it a mandate for receiving certain blessings. While we may wonder why it took them so long, consider how well our generation is doing at keeping the rest of the counsel in the Word of Wisdom without an unambiguous mandate to do so. According to a study done at Brigham Young University, LDS college students are generally quite familiar with the positive aspects of the Word of Wisdom, but the gap between what they *believe* they should do and what they actually *do* is enormous.[15] As my cousin puts it, "The Mormon culture is still pretty meat-and-treat heavy." Studies indicate "LDS meat consumption to be as high or higher than national averages."[16] And statistics show that Utah Mormons are "significantly heavier" than Utah non-Mormons.[17] This is sad evidence supporting the accusation that we are *fatter*-day saints.

We have been given the Word of Wisdom to guide our actions, and our leaders have left us to decide how we will respond. I'm glad the Church has clarified that we should not consume illicit drugs, alcohol, and tobacco. When I think of how much heartache and devastating health consequences this has spared us, I am grateful beyond words! If the Church had not been so clear on this, my guess is that many of us, like the early Saints, would choose the route of "moderation." But why settle for a *moderate* amount of the blessings?

I personally do not believe the positive admonitions of the Word of Wisdom will ever be mandated by the Church. Nor do I think they need to be mandated in order for us to benefit from them. If we as Latter-day Saints were not falling victim to the devastating chronic illnesses found in the general population, we might be forgiven for ignoring them. While we truly have been greatly blessed by avoiding many harmful substances, most of us will at some point still fall victim to serious health problems that could have been avoided had we understood and followed the truths found in the Word of Wisdom. Let us, instead, lay claim to all of the blessings the Lord is pleased to give us.

## LDS Leaders on the Word of Wisdom

With all the work it took early Church leaders to finally get the Saints to give up the use of alcohol, tobacco, coffee, and tea, I am not surprised that no more effort has been put into emphasizing other aspects of the Word of Wisdom. Nevertheless, throughout the Church's history, leaders have spoken on many aspects of the Word of Wisdom beyond the prohibited substances.[18] In this section, I'll mention a few I especially like.

The Prophet Joseph Smith's beloved brother, Hyrum Smith, was Patriarch to the Church when he delivered a beautiful address on the Word of Wisdom in 1842. The following is but a small part of his much longer exhortation on this topic:

> [God] knows what course to pursue to restore mankind to their pristine excellency and primitive vigor, and health; and he has appointed the word of wisdom as one of the engines to bring about this thing, to remove the beastly appetites, the murderous disposition and the vitiated taste of man; to restore his body to health, and vigour, promote peace between him and the brute creation. . . .
>
> Let men attend to [the Word of Wisdom], let them use the things ordained of God; let them be sparing of the life of animals; 'it is pleasing saith the Lord that flesh be used only in times of winter, or of famine'—and why to be used in famine? because all domesticated animals would naturally die, and may as well be made use of by man, as not.[19]

In 1897, before he became prophet, Apostle Lorenzo Snow spoke with the First Presidency and other Apostles on the subject of the Word of Wisdom,

> expressing the opinion that it was violated as much or more in the improper use of meat as in other things, and thought the time was near at hand when the Latter Day Saints should be taught to refrain from meat eating and the shedding of animal blood.[20]

A year later, he spoke again to his brethren on the Word of Wisdom:

> [He] drew special attention to that part which relates to the use of meats, which he considered just as strong as that which relates to the use of liquors and hot drinks. He also referred to the revelation which says that he that forbids the use of meat is not of God.... Bro. Snow said he was convinced that the killing of animals when unnecessary was wrong and sinful, and that it was not right to neglect one part of the Word of Wisdom and be too strenuous in regard to other parts.[21]

In a 1948 General Conference address entitled "Eat Flesh Sparingly," Elder Joseph F. Merrill focused specifically on the consumption of meat:

> All over the Church the belief is general that the Word of Wisdom is practically observed if the individual abstains from the use of tea, coffee, liquor, and tobacco. But a careful reading of the revelation shows this belief to be erroneous. There is much more to the document than abstention from the use of narcotics. ... According to what are regarded as the best investigations, the right proportion of protein is generally about 10 percent of the total number of heat units consumed. ... The foods to be used most sparingly are those which contain a great excess of protein, such as meat, eggs, cheese, and beans. On this account, there are many authorities who think that it would be safer to discard the use of meat altogether than to continue to use it so freely as many Americans are doing.[22]

In a 1979 address to the BYU community, Elder Ezra Taft Benson counseled:

> There is no question that the health of the body affects the spirit, or the Lord would never have revealed the Word of Wisdom. ... To a great extent we are physically what we eat. Most of us are acquainted with some of the prohibitions, such as no tea, coffee, tobacco, or alcohol. What needs additional emphasis are the positive aspects—the need for vegetables, fruits, and grains, particularly wheat. In most cases, the closer these can be, when eaten, to their natural state—without over refinement and processing—the healthier we will be. To a significant degree, we are an overfed and undernourished nation

digging an early grave with our teeth, and lacking the energy
that could be ours because we overindulge in junk foods. . . .
We need a generation of young people who, as Daniel, eat in
a more healthy manner than to fare on the "king's meat"—
and whose countenances show it (see Daniel 1).[23]

Elder Gordon B. Hinckley spoke often on the Word of Wisdom, encouraging members to live it more carefully. During the 1990 General
Conference, he noted that the Word of Wisdom "proscribes alcohol and
tobacco, tea and coffee, and emphasizes the use of fruit and grains." He
added, "This Word of Wisdom came to us from the God of Heaven, for
our blessing. I regret that we as a people do not observe it more faithfully."[24] Again in 1993, he said:

I thank the Lord for a testimony of the Word of Wisdom. I
wish we lived it more fully. But even though we do not, the
Lord pours out His blessings upon those who try.[25]

Many more Church leaders have spoken out on aspects of this revelation beyond the prohibitions. Instead of asking, "Why they don't tell us
more?" I now find myself wondering, "Why haven't I listened better?"

## LDS Leaders, Leading by Example

At least a few of our latter-day prophets made the personal decision in
their own diet to emphasize the positive aspects of the Word of Wisdom,
including eating very little meat.

No modern-day prophet was a greater champion for the Word of Wisdom than President Heber J. Grant. He lived the Word of Wisdom and
attributed his excellent health, in part, to eating very little meat. In the
1937 General Conference, at 80 years old, he said he worked long hours
"without fatigue and without feeling the least injury." He explained:

I think that another reason why I have very splendid strength
for an old man is that during the years we have had a caf-
eteria in the Utah Hotel, I have not, with the exception of
not more than a dozen times, ordered meat of any kind. On
these special occasions I have mentioned I have perhaps had
a small, tender lamb chop. I have endeavored to live the Word
of Wisdom, and that, in my opinion, is one reason for my
good health.[26]

President George Albert Smith was also careful about his consumption of meat. In the 1950 *Improvement Era* devoted to honoring his 80th birthday, his son-in-law reported:

> President Smith's meals are simple and nourishing. In the summer he eats no meat, and even in the winter months he eats very little.[27]

President Joseph Fielding Smith, like his father Joseph F. Smith, often expressed concern for animals, believing them to be eternal creatures that would be resurrected to a state of glory.[28] In 1970, his wife, Jessie Evans Smith, reported, "My husband doesn't eat meat. . . . We eat lots of fruits and vegetables."[29]

President Ezra Taft Benson's son said that his father, "In his personal life, was sparing in his use of meat and generous in his use of fresh vegetables and grains."[30]

In an unforgettable 1978 General Conference, President Spencer W. Kimball shared cherished songs from his youth including *In Our Lovely Deseret*, penned by Eliza R. Snow. He quoted this lovely pioneer hymn, which includes the words:

> That the children may live long
> And be beautiful and strong,
> Tea and coffee and tobacco they despise,
> Drink no liquor, and they eat
> *But a very little meat;*
> They are seeking to be great and good and wise.
> (LDS Hymn #307, emphasis added)

Immediately after sharing line five, President Kimball interjected, "I still don't eat very much meat."[31] He went on in this address and in the next Conference to share his "feelings concerning the unnecessary shedding of blood and destruction of [animal] life."[32]

Eating is a social activity. It is not easy to make dietary changes that are out of step with family, friends, and society, especially for men who may not prepare most of their own food. Yet these men did not wait for an official Church pronouncement to try to adjust their diet to be more in harmony with the wisdom of D&C 89. Nor as prophets did they mandate that all Church members make the same decision. We are each left to decide how we wish to interpret and implement the counsel in Section 89.

# Real Mormons ❧ Real Stories

## *Jessica's Story*

My parents raised me on a fairly healthy diet: lots of fruits and vegetables and little sugar. However, that does not always mean a person has a healthy attitude. I did experiment with vegetarianism and veganism at several different points through high school, but I thought of it as another diet and never stuck to it—the moment my dad made barbeque chicken, that was it!

Shortly after getting married, I found myself sitting in a Relief Society class discussing the Word of Wisdom. It was a very interesting lesson to me, and I listened closely to my sisters' opinions on what it said, and how we can eat healthy based on its principles. I skimmed over Section 89 as everyone else talked, and my eyes lighted on something:

> Yea, flesh also of beasts and of the fowls of the air, I, the Lord, have ordained for the use of man with thanksgiving; nevertheless they are to be used sparingly; And it is pleasing unto me that they should not be used, only in times of winter, or of cold, or famine. (D&C 89:12–13)

I blinked at these words and looked around at the rest of the class. Why had no one brought these verses up? They were all discussing alcohol, tea, tobacco, fruits, and vegetables, these two verses forgotten. To me, it seemed clear: God didn't want us to eat meat unless strictly necessary for survival.

I came home from church that afternoon and told my husband (over beef roast) about the thoughts I'd had on the Word of Wisdom during class, and how I wanted to start eating less meat right away. He agreed with how I felt, and we agreed to stop buying meat.

The two of us began to evaluate the rest of our diet, quickly eliminating all processed foods as well. At this point I said, "Hey, you know what? I'm sleeping better. But the Word of Wisdom promises that we'll run and not be weary, and walk and not faint—I think there's something we're still doing wrong in our diet."

"Could be," my husband said, and we began to pray fervently for the answer to 100% complete health.

Then I got pregnant, and all our accomplishments in the last few months became harder. I was sick all the time, and the only things I could think of eating that wouldn't make me throw up were (processed) crackers, (sugar-filled) popsicles, and (chicken) broth. I took a new stand: anything that sounded edible, I ate.

The baby was born. I continued to eat the way we'd eaten during the pregnancy. This wasn't strictly bad, but there were several processed items in our diet, not to mention meat.

I was dropping weight like crazy thanks to the breastfeeding, and I began to get obsessed with the weight I could lose. Then my husband pointed out that I was losing my healthy attitude about food. I realized he was right, and renewed my prayers to know the healthiest way to eat.

I decided to study the matter more scientifically, rather than relying on the scriptures alone: I got on Amazon and searched for books on health. *The China Study* was third most popular, and seemed the most promising, so I immediately bought it as an e-book and began to read.

I wasn't even past the introduction when I realized this wasn't just any health book—this book was advocating what I personally recognized as veganism. Veganism—one step further than the vegetarianism advocated by the Word of Wisdom. Could eliminating milk be the missing puzzle piece to full health? And then I felt the rush of the Spirit—I was still in the introduction—and knew I would take everything Dr. Campbell said seriously.

As I continued to read, everything made sense. I knew this was the answer I'd been looking for, the answer to getting my health as close to 100% as possible.

My husband, who had previously given up meat so easily, was convinced dairy was necessary. That's when my new ideas became more difficult—if he didn't support this, how could I make it happen? But I knew the Spirit had confirmed this path, and so I strode forward faithfully, relying on science most of the time, and relying on the Spirit when those arguments felt weak.

My headaches went away within two weeks. My menstrual cycle became ridiculously easy to handle compared to before. I had so much energy to chase my son around!

After a few months, my husband and I sat down and watched the *Forks Over Knives* documentary together. That night he leaned over on the couch, kissed me, and said, "Thank you." It was one of the happiest moments of my life.

My biggest difficultly was in what I was going to give my son instead of cow's milk. Eventually, after watching him, I realized that he was taking care of it himself. I provided healthy options, and he told me what he wanted—and he began to grow like crazy!

We still face difficulties, but we have found good solutions to all major problems: family reunions, restaurants, social events. Most people at church don't know about our lifestyle, but the ones who care do, and hopefully that'll make a difference to them.

Best of all, my body does exactly what it's supposed to. My weight is managing itself for the most part, and I've found the joy of plants. Beyond the physical benefits, my testimony is stronger than it ever has been because I've learned to rely on the Spirit for everything I need in life—especially how to physically care for myself and my family. I've never been happier and more energetic!

*Jessica Knutson and her husband have one son. They currently reside in Springville, Utah, but are off to Oregon in the spring. She earned her BA in History and is now trying to get a fictional book published while her toddler sleeps.*

# 10

# The Promised Blessings

The Word of Wisdom was explicitly given as "A principle with promise" (D&C 89:3). Before even mentioning the wonderful spiritual promises, the physical blessings are staggering. If members of the Church voluntarily chose to adhere strictly to the counsel in the Word of Wisdom, the evidence suggests we would virtually eliminate the chronic diseases this revelation seems custom-designed to combat, and many other diseases would be reduced dramatically. We would quickly become the single largest, healthiest population in the United States. The difference would be so dramatic, others would take notice, and we would have the opportunity to share this beautiful health message with them, opening additional opportunities for spreading the gospel. Other blessings we would receive are too numerous to specify, but just one example: literally thousands, if not tens of thousands and eventually millions, more LDS senior couples would have the strength and vitality to serve missions, even multiple missions, for the Church. This is just one way we could play a greater role in the Lord's effort to hasten His work in these last days.

The blessings promised by the Lord in the Word of Wisdom are breathtaking:

> And all saints who remember to keep and do these sayings, walking in obedience to the commandments, shall receive health in their navel and marrow to their bones;
>
> And shall find wisdom and great treasures of knowledge, even hidden treasures;

And shall run and not be weary, and shall walk and not faint.

And I, the Lord, give unto them a promise, that the destroying angel shall pass by them, as the children of Israel, and not slay them. Amen. (D&C 89:18–21)

I am filled with gratitude to the Lord every time I read these promises and consider how much He desires to bless us. As an apostle, Harold B. Lee said the following about the promise of protection implied in the last verse:

There are promises of protection in the Word of Wisdom. The Lord's word of wisdom commanding abstinence from a worldly "king's portion" of tobacco, tea and coffee, and alcoholic beverages that are habit-forming, and which counsels the simple diet of fruits, grains, and vegetables in season, with meats used sparingly, has been given you as a revelation of God's great law of health. It stands today as a challenge to a world surfeited with things condemned as unclean and unfit for the human body. If you have faith as the youthful Daniel and his brethren and purpose in your hearts that you will not defile yourselves with "king's meat and wine," even though you may be two thousand miles east of the Suez Canal, your faith will have the reward of hidden treasures of knowledge, of strong bodies that can "run and not be weary and walk and not faint." If by faith in this great law, you refrain from the use of food and drink harmful to your bodies, you will not become a ready prey to scourges that shall sweep the land, as in the days of the people of Moses in Egypt, bringing death to every household that has not heeded the commandments of God.[1]

I want to repeat that last sentence because it is now clear how prophetic Elder Lee's words were:

If by faith in this great law, you refrain from the use of food and drink harmful to your bodies, *you will not become a ready prey to scourges that shall sweep the land, as in the days of the people of Moses in Egypt, bringing death to every household that has not heeded the commandments of God.*

We now see that the way we are eating is indeed "bringing death to [almost] every household" as we find people around us succumbing to illnesses that are virtually 100 percent preventable by strict adherence to the Word of Wisdom. Are there not already scourges of heart disease, cancer, obesity, and diabetes that are sweeping our land? And who is to say when the prophecies will come to pass and we "shall see an overflowing scourge; for a desolating sickness shall cover the land" (D&C 45:31). Whether it is incurable superbugs or other threatening diseases, when God warns the inhabitants of the earth by spreading "pestilences of every kind" (D&C 43:25), will not our obedience to the Word of Wisdom protect us? Will we not be grateful for the Lord's promise "that the destroying angel shall pass by [us], as the children of Israel, and not slay [us]" (D&C 89:21)?

Elder George Q. Cannon warned in 1892:

> Our religion impresses upon us the importance of taking care of our bodies. Yet, notwithstanding that which the Lord has done for us in revealing to us the true principles of life, there is a great amount of ignorance even among us upon this important subject. . . . Many of the Saints do not seem to be alive to the importance of those laws which pertain to well-being and preservation of the health and strength of the body. Their old traditions cling to them, and it appears to be difficult for them to shake them off. Yet the day must come when the people of God will be superiors physically and mentally, to every other people upon the face of the earth. Before this day shall come . . . pestilence of various kinds, which we are led to expect through the word of the Lord are yet to break forth, will have their effect in calling the Saints' attention to those laws of life and health which, to be a strong and vigorous people, we must observe.
>
> If pestilence should stalk through the land . . . many who are now careless respecting the words of the Lord contained in the Word of Wisdom will be likely to reform their habits and pay attention to the counsels which He there gives. . . . We are promised greater safety than other people are likely to enjoy; but the promises are based on certain conditions, which must be observed . . . why should people in our day expect to enjoy health and an exemption from the visit of the destroyer when he goes forth as he did in Egypt if they do not comply with the conditions which the Lord has prescribed.[2]

I certainly feel I have been blessed by following a diet more in harmony with the Word of Wisdom than what I used to eat. I mentioned that I lost weight: 25 pounds in less than a year. I'm now back to the weight I was when I graduated from high school. Along with the pounds, all of the other small health problems that had developed over the years have also disappeared. My biomarkers are all excellent. I have lots of energy, and I feel great!

I have not entirely avoided ill health, however. I've had two nasty colds since I started the diet, but I count both as blessings. They were vivid reminders that I'd so much rather enjoy my delicious WFPB diet than invite more ill health, much less chronic disease!

When I started this diet it was the physical benefits that most attracted me, that most thrilled me. But over time other benefits began to outweigh the physical ones and have become much more precious. Now I realize that the rich abundance of sweet spiritual blessings I have experienced far exceed the physical ones. While I have focused almost exclusively on the temporal blessings of obeying the Word of Wisdom in this book, clearly the spiritual blessings are most important, and these blessings have been the ones most emphasized by LDS Church leaders. Elder Stephen L. Richards taught:

> Every commandment of God is spiritual in nature.... While the commandments have effect upon the body and temporal things they are all in essence spiritual. The Word of Wisdom is spiritual. It is true that it enjoins the use of deleterious substances and makes provision for the health of the body. But the largest measure of good derived from its observance is in increased faith and the development of more spiritual power and wisdom. Likewise, the most regrettable and damaging effects of its infractions are spiritual, also.[3]

In the October 2013 General Conference, Elder Russell M. Nelson reminded us that our bodies are a "vital part of God's eternal plan." He taught that the decisions we make in how we care for our bodies will "determine your destiny" because "your body is the temple for your spirit. And how you use your body affects your spirit."[4]

I testify that the blessings of living the Word of Wisdom are both physical and spiritual. The Lord is true to His word. If we heed His counsel, He will bestow the blessings of the Word of Wisdom on us. I now know this from personal experience in ways I did not know when I only kept part of the Word of Wisdom. President Boyd K. Packer taught, "The Word of Wisdom is a key to individual revelation."[5] As we purify our physical tabernacles, we invite the Spirit of God to dwell with us more fully, which leads to discovering "wisdom and great treasures of knowledge, even hidden treasures" (D&C 89:19). I would not trade the rich spiritual treasures I've received by keeping the Word of Wisdom for all the wealth of the world. No one can convince me now that the Standard American Diet is worth the price we pay. It is a mess of pottage—worse, in fact, since real pottage is much more nutritious.

While I certainly do not believe I will never have any health problems or that others following this diet will eliminate all health issues, I do believe anyone observing the advice in Section 89 will receive unmistakable physical and spiritual blessings. We have the Lord's promise.

## Eating as a Sanctifying Experience

In writing this book, I have learned a great many new things. Every time I thought the book was complete, a new vista opened up for my consideration, and I had to add a new section. This section of the book is no different. I thought I was finished. I was reading through the materials I had collected to make sure I had not missed anything when I discovered I had missed something: a short article I had by BYU professor of Church History, Paul H. Peterson, "The Sanctity of Food: A Latter-day Saint Perspective," first published in 2001.[6]

I was already acquainted with Paul Peterson's 1972 BYU Master's thesis, the first (and in many ways still the best) comprehensive historical analysis ever done on the Word of Wisdom. In this thesis, Peterson specifically states he will address only the prohibitions in the Word of Wisdom. In one of the few references he makes to those who would "broaden" the meaning of Word of Wisdom, he links such people with "extremists" and "food faddists" who are "out of line with Church policy" (p. 100). It seemed clear he had little interest in these other aspects. Apparently, that attitude changed at some point in his life.

Though the Word of Wisdom was not the focus of his scholarship throughout his lifetime, Petersen did write occasionally on the topic. At the conclusion of his long career, while serving as chair of the BYU Church History and Doctrine Department, he published "The Sanctity of Food," an article which I now believe I was meant to read and include in this book.

In this work, Petersen describes the "sanctifying sense" many observant Jewish people have toward food and the way their approach to diet helps make "everyday life [become] nobler and purer" (p. 33). He laments that the Latter-day Saints do not have the same attitude toward eating. While we believe the body is sacred, eating is a means to an end for most of us. He goes on to summarize the history of the Word of Wisdom and questions why the focus for LDS members has been on the *proscriptions* rather than the *prescriptions*. He asks why Latter-day Saints have paid so little attention to the positive aspects of the Word of Wisdom, those that might actually make eating a more "sanctifying" experience. He then makes an astonishing prediction:

> Although the differences and distinctions between Latter-day Saint and Jewish attitudes to food and diet will probably always be greater than the similarities, it is possible that in the future, many Latter-day Saints, of their own volition, will adopt attitudes and assume patterns toward food and drink that are somewhat analogous to the Jewish approach. I predict (some would say, with unwarranted temerity) that some alteration of attitudes will take place along two fronts. The first such front has to do with the broadening of Word of Wisdom considerations to include more than just the present list of proscriptions. *In short, in all likelihood, more and more Latter-day Saints will come to view Doctrine and Covenants 89 not only as a delineator of forbidden items but also as an indicator of what one should eat.* (p. 39, emphasis added)

I was stunned when I read these words. I suddenly realized that my experience in changing my diet and helping other Saints to do the same was a literal fulfillment of Peterson's prediction.

Peterson goes on to discuss the reasons these changes might take place. Most of these I have already covered in this book, including "strong scriptural precedents—both in canonized scripture and in the statements of presiding brethren" (p. 40). He describes the second reason this change may occur is that LDS views on stewardship to the earth and animals is very compatible with a Word of Wisdom approach to "environmental sensitivity and holistic living" (p. 40). He concludes:

> Clearly then, there are both scriptural and prophetic precedents for members of the Church—if they so desire to expand their own personal list of Word of Wisdom considerations. There are also scriptural and prophetic models for

viewing the entire revelation in a more holistic way . . . by our viewing the eating of foods that God has prescribed as a spiritual act or event. (p. 41)

Peterson suggests that like observant Jews, Latter-day Saints can, "by eating some foods and refraining from others in obedience to their religion, actually elevate the act of eating to a level of godliness" (p. 42). He explains:

> Although such a view is hardly widespread in the Latter-day Saint community, it is scripturally supportable. For example, why couldn't Latter-day Saints, by avoiding the food and drink God has placed off limits and by eating only those foods they believe God has singled out as being especially good for mankind, gain greater reverence for life and increased appreciation for the Lord? My suspicion is that in the future, some Church members will do so and thus come to regard eating as much more than just a practical necessity. (p. 42)

How might it change the way we eat if we viewed the everyday practice of preparing and consuming food as part of our worship of God?

Finally, Peterson concludes with an observation that is just beginning to help me see what I am doing in a whole different light: he observes that a similarity between Latter-day Saints and observant Jews is that our dietary codes are central to our identity, both as individuals and as a community. The Word of Wisdom is, after all, one of the most identifying features of our religion from the perspective of nonmembers.[7] It is one of the features that set us apart as a people. All observant Latter-day Saints experience this distinction when they are in a group of non-Latter-day Saints. Food is so central to who we are as humans that the fact that we do not partake of certain substances almost always becomes apparent when we mix with others not of our faith. It sets us apart. It reminds others, and it reminds us, of who we are.

For observant Jews, their dietary laws are, in the words of Jewish author Herman Wouk, "a daily commitment in action to one's faith, a formal choice, a quiet self-discipline" (p. 43). Peterson concludes:

> Possibly to a lesser but still a highly meaningful extent, the Word of Wisdom has served a similar function among Latter-day Saints. Every time a Church member politely says

"no thank you" to the generous offer of an acquaintance or stranger to partake of coffee or alcohol, the action has the effect of reminding everyone involved that Latter-day Saints are a "separate people," that they made covenants with the Lord, and that because of their "peculiarity," there are things they can and cannot do. Indeed, it is difficult to conceive of a more suitable vehicle to remind us of our covenantal responsibilities and embed them into our self-consciousness than to require certain patterns of eating and drinking—something that is usually done openly and daily. (p. 43)

We often think of the Word of Wisdom as a "health code," but it serves many other purposes, including reminding us of the covenants we have made with the Lord, giving us an opportunity to obey Him in the simple mundane things we do every day, and setting us apart as a people. We actually don't know which of the many purposes ultimately will be most important to us, either as individuals or as a community, but it is beautiful to me to realize that the every day act of nourishing our bodies can be a sanctifying experience.

## Waking Up to the Word of Wisdom

As Peterson points out, the community or *social* aspect of keeping the Word of Wisdom can't be avoided. There is no doubt that the most difficult part of adopting a WFPB diet is the social aspect. Food is integral to who we are, not just as individuals, but most importantly as a community. Food is a social event, and when we eat differently than others, it can be extremely awkward and uncomfortable.

I have certainly experienced this awkwardness during the past two years. I find my new diet sometimes sets me apart from other people. This is an issue every person who changes his or her diet must negotiate. For many, it is not easy. I remind people who are facing these challenges that they are pioneers. Like new converts to the Church, their family and friends may not understand or approve of what they are doing. Some may scold or mock. Others may just feel uncomfortable. Even in a supportive environment, it is difficult to eat differently, if for logistical reasons alone.

I try to remind those who are changing their diet that while it is not easy to be a pioneer, it is important. It is important for our health, and it is important for the health of those we love. Even if others do not know it, they likely need this diet. When the day comes that they long for better health, they will be able to turn to the pioneers they know for help. They will remember the way the diet helped us gain better health and will learn how to claim the same blessings for themselves.

Before stumbling on to the WFPB diet, I had no desire to become a pioneer or any kind of a Word of Wisdom missionary. I was not seeking to change how I ate. I did not have serious health issues diet could address. Finding this diet was literally an answer to a question I did not have. But for many reasons, it resonated with me. One reason was my long familiarity with the Word of Wisdom. I remember reading Section 89 soon after learning about this diet and delighting in how perfectly they seemed to match. Between the scientific reasoning and this revelation from God, I was convinced that this is the diet we humans are supposed to be eating. I felt elated.

I also felt full of desire to share this treasure with other people. I didn't actually think anyone else would be crazy enough to give up their fat-saturated, sweet, scrumptious food, but I was wrong. As I share this diet with my fellow Latter-day Saints, people are very receptive. It seems to resonate with them as well. I've now personally shared this diet through mostly one-on-one conversations with hundreds of people. Most of them have expressed some degree of interest, and dozens of them have changed their diet, many quite dramatically. I think one reason the diet resonates with them is their familiarity with the Word of Wisdom. Now, in writing this book, and specifically in collecting stories from other people, I see that Mormons in all walks of life are discovering the Word of Wisdom, just as I am. There must be a reason for this great awakening.

For over 15 years I've worked at Brigham Young University in faculty development. As part of my job, we organize dozens of faculty workshops and seminars each year. Because we often have meals at these seminars and I eat with the faculty participants, I have had to figure out how to both do my job and stay on my new diet. Fortunately, BYU Catering has come through with flying colors, preparing many delicious plant-based meals for me. Of course, others sometimes notice my food is different and ask me about it. Rather than be embarrassed, I use this opportunity to very briefly tell them why I changed my diet and how enthused I am about it. Because I'd never want to imply that anyone who does not eat like this is not obeying the Word of Wisdom, I've rarely mentioned it, but others make the connection themselves and sometimes bring it up in our conversation. Most are at least curious, others quite interested, and there are consistently a few who would "like to know more." It is always a thrill to share what I know with those who are interested, and provide them with a few resources to help them on their journey.

In our work at the BYU Faculty Center we use a database to keep track of the faculty members we serve, so I turned to this source to get a few basic facts about Paul Peterson for this book. There were several facts listed, but the one that made me smile was the note we had taken of his dietary preference: "Vegetarian." It is interesting that even the scholar who, very early in his career, wrote perhaps the best history of the Word of Wisdom was, at the end of his career, still waking up to the Word of Wisdom.

## Hidden Treasures

I am grateful for modern medicine, including the appropriate use of drugs and surgery. I do not believe even the best nutrition solves every health issue. I finally did have a total hip replacement in January 2012 and a second one in December 2012. I am *very hip* now, and I love it! These surgeries did for me what perfect nutrition could not have done: eliminated the pain of two congenitally deformed hips.

It is not in God's plan that we never suffer. I believe we can learn things from physical pain and illness that we cannot learn in any other way. One of the precious truths I learned through my experience with hip pain is that *this mortal life is the only time in all of eternity where we can learn those things we can only learn through physical pain and suffering.* Nevertheless, not all suffering is necessary, and the Lord has a vested interest in the health of His Saints. He cares about our health and what we eat. One of the first commandments given to Adam and Eve had to do with what they should and should not eat. He gave the children of Israel dietary laws that fit their circumstances. And as part of the Restoration and in preparation for the last days, He has given us the Word of Wisdom.

The Word of Wisdom blessed me even before my entry into this world because my parents kept it (as they understood it) and therefore allowed my body to develop in a womb that was free from all kinds of harmful substances. I was taught the Word of Wisdom from birth through the examples of my parents, grandparents, and other family members who lived by many of its precepts. I'm sure I was taught the Word of Wisdom as a child many times before my first memories of it happening. I have always known the basics of the Word of Wisdom, and that it is essential for us to follow. I've sat through countless lessons on the Word of Wisdom as a child, as a teenager, as a young adult, and even now as an adult I continue to be taught about the Word of Wisdom on Sundays and through Church magazines and other media.

Because the Word of Wisdom has always been part of my life, I am amazed to still be learning there is so much more to this treasured document. There are many more blessings the Lord would like to give us through adherence to its principles than I ever imagined. And consider, this precious health code is the stripped-down "adapted" version: "adapted to the capacity of the weak, and the weakest of all saints" (D&C 89:3). What does the full health code look like? And what will be the blessings of obeying it?

All of this makes me wonder what other principles with a promise are scattered throughout the scriptures, just waiting for us to recognize and act on them? What wisdom and hidden treasures do we pass by? Do we need to have Church leaders point each out unambiguously before we act on them? I think Church leaders have their hands full trying to help us recognize and act on the most important, basic, and fundamental principles of the gospel. These are the foundations, but the Lord has more in store for us, more blessings, more promises. What is to keep us from seeking these also?

I rejoice in the hope that my understanding of God's revelations will continue to grow and expand. I know I have much to learn, and I welcome any insights others reading this book would like to share. Thank you!

## Real Mormons ❧ Real Stories

### Karen's Story

In the summer of 2011 Border's Books was going out of business so I decided to see if there were some books that might interest me. I gravitated toward the health section and picked up a book called *The China Study* by T. Colin Campbell. My husband's cousin, a doctor, had recently mentioned this book in a Facebook post, and I was curious about it.

During this same summer, my sister-in-law was living with us while she had radiation treatments for breast cancer. My husband was working out of town and our children were all grown and out of the house, so my sister-in-law and I were the only ones at home. Because of her cancer, she was taking a greater interest in getting proper nutrition. Her doctor had told her "to not eat any dairy as it promotes tumor growth." She was buying organic fruits and vegetables and trying new healthy recipes.

I was interested in eating healthier too. I was nearly 50 years old. I had slowly gained 35 lbs over 30 years of marriage. Several friends my age and younger were being diagnosed with breast cancer. It seemed so random. I also noticed many of our friends who were a decade older were starting to experience a lot of health problems.

I began reading *The China Study* and was immediately hit with a strong feeling that what I was reading was true. As I read, I felt compelled on several occasions to open up the Doctrine and Covenants and read Section 89. Each time I did, I was struck with the realization that the Lord, our Creator, was recommending a diet of plant-based whole foods, which was the same thing I was reading about in *The China Study*. Why had I not seen or understood this before? I don't know why, but now I knew the kind of foods I should be eating, and I knew I had to make a change. I also felt a sense of peace when I learned there were actually things I could do to help prevent many of the common and most prevalent cancers—breast, colon, ovarian—as well as many chronic diseases like heart disease, stroke (which my grandfather had), high blood pressure, kidney disease, diabetes, and Alzheimer's disease (which my grandmother had).

As I began to think about changing the way I eat, I felt a panicky feeling. What would I eat? What would I fix for dinner? What would my husband say? What would my children say? What would I do when I was invited to eat at someone's home? I didn't know the answers to these questions, but I decided to have faith in the Lord and trust that it would all be OK.

I began searching the Internet for recipes. I went back to Border's and purchased vegetarian cookbooks. I started trying new recipes and discovered some really fantastic ones! Within a very short period of time, my taste buds changed. I LOVED the foods I was eating! Fruit tasted so sweet. I felt as if my taste buds had woken up and become alive, the new flavors were so delicious to me!

Also, I felt so good eating these foods! I have a hard time describing it, but after I would eat a meal of plant-based whole foods, I would feel this wonderful feeling from inside. Once in a while, in the beginning, I "cheated" a little. I noticed I did not have this wonderful feeling inside on those occasions. It was as if there was instant positive reinforcement each time I ate these marvelous foods, and I felt so excited I had stumbled upon this amazing new way to eat. Another thing I really loved about this way of eating is that I could eat a lot of food and not worry about counting calories ever again. I could eat until I was comfortably full and then when I got hungry I could eat again. I realized it was something I could do for the rest of my life.

As I mentioned previously, I had gained 35 lbs during the previous 30 years, and I didn't like how I looked or how I felt. About two years before changing my diet, I started exercising on a regular basis and trying to eat "healthier." In addition to the exercise, I also started counting calories. I competed in four sprint triathlons that year. I lost about 27 lbs but then regained about 13 lbs, even though I was extremely active and was training for a century bike ride (a 100 mile bike ride). I decided my current weight of 145 lbs was probably where I was going to stay. My height is 5'7", and I thought that it was a pretty good weight for my height.

When I began eating plant-based whole foods, the extra weight fell off effortlessly and eventually stabilized at 125 lbs, which is what I weighed when I got married at 19 years old. I have kept the weight off with no problem these past two years. I also noticed my headaches went away. I used to get headaches fairly often, and now I get one maybe once every few months. My cholesterol was at 159, which isn't bad, but it dropped to 118. When I discovered I was losing weight without even trying, I thought to myself, "I have discovered the secret to weight loss everyone has been looking for!!!!" I was sad to realize most people didn't want to even consider this way of eating as a way to lose weight and regain their health.

As I mentioned, my husband was working out of town when I started this diet. He worked 28 days out of town, would come home for four or five days, and then leave again for 28 days and so on. When he came home one day from one of his trips, I said, "Honey, guess what? I no longer eat meat or dairy or other foods that aren't healthy. I'm eating a whole new way now." I was worried how he would react to this news. After all, we had been married 30 years at this point, and he was used to me cooking all the meals. He was surprisingly supportive, I think because I was losing weight and he liked the change and didn't want to mess that up!

I would experiment with new recipes while my husband was out of town and then when he was home, I'd cook him the best ones. He liked the foods I was preparing for our meals. I had high hopes that he would want to change too but now, two years later, he still likes to eat the Standard American Diet. He eats the food I prepare for him, but when he goes out to eat, he orders the typical food like he always has. I try not to criticize his food choices or nag him about eating better, as that would only cause contention. My husband is no longer working out of town and is back at home full-time. I'm really happy about that, and he is still pleased as can be that his wife has the figure she did 30 years ago when he married her!

I am not tempted to go back to my old way of eating because I feel so great! I have more energy, I sleep well, and I can easily maintain my weight. I have never felt so much joy over food . . . I just love it so much! I don't have to clean up greasy dishes anymore, and I feel at peace knowing I can do something to prevent many of the common chronic illnesses that plague our society.

*Karen Barnes, age 52, lives in Gilbert, Arizona where she is the owner of a custom drapery manufacturing business. Outside of work, she enjoys spending time with family and is an avid cyclist. She and her husband have four children and eight grandchildren.*

# Appendix 1

## *More* Real Mormons Real Stories

Writing this book introduced me to many Latter-day Saints who are discovering the Word of Wisdom. I love knowing that Mormons of all ages and in all walks of life are being inspired to live a whole food, plant-based lifestyle. I am grateful they are willing to share their stories with us. You can see photos of these authors, along with many more stories, on the website discoveringthewordofwisdom.com. I hope you will be willing to share your story when you are ready!

- **Children**
    - Sally, Elaine, and Mariah George
- **Pre-Teens**
    - Bradshaw Hirschi
    - Shayne Hirschi
- **Teens**
    - Liesel Allen
    - Michael Anderson
- **The 20's**
    - Victor Johnson
    - Robyn Rowley
- **The 30's**
    - Christie Cosky
    - Charity Lighten

- **The 40's**
    - Laura Bridgewater
    - Kevin Tunstall
- **The 50's**
    - Orva Johnson
    - Elna Clark
- **The 60's**
    - Christine Bradley
    - Tim and Ellen McGaughy
- **The 70's**
    - Sandra Cherry
- **The 80's**
    - Neil Birch

# Children

Heavenly Father wants us to eat bread and peas and cantaloupe. And we can eat pineapple and white beans. We should not eat cheese.

We don't eat meat because meat is not good for us. It has sugar in it, maybe? My favorite thing to eat is peas, carrots, and cucumbers with hummus. I also like raw cinnamon rolls, snack bars, sweet potato fries, and kale chips.

I wish I could eat the treats in my nursery class. I should tell them it has sugar in it, and they could do a puzzle instead.

*Sally George is 3 and lives in Oklahoma. She loves to take care of her babies, ride her bike, and eat.*

We are vegan so that we don't get cancer and so we don't get sick. The Lord wants us to eat things that are healthy. The Word of Wisdom says to not eat cows.

My favorite things to eat are beans, rice, and corn, enchiladas, barbeque tofu pizza, grilled cheez, and quesadilla [all made without dairy!]. The hardest part of being vegan is I really like candy, and I don't get to usually eat it. I'm glad we're vegan because I don't like cheese, and I wouldn't like chicken and ham! I will be vegan when I grow up.

*Elaine George is 5 and lives in Oklahoma. She loves to play with play-doh, go to pre-k, and dance.*

We are vegan because my grandpa got diabetes, and my grandma found out it was because of too much meat and dairy. Heavenly Father wants us to eat grains, fruit, and vegetables. I feel good when I follow the Word of Wisdom. My favorite meal is hashbrowns and French toast made with tofu instead of eggs.

When it is red ribbon week [a drug prevention campaign], I will tell my teacher that in my church, we don't drink hot drinks such as tea and coffee—even grown-ups don't do it! And I hope they are happy to hear that!

*Mariah George is 6 and lives in Oklahoma. She loves to draw, dance, and read.*

# Pre-Teens

I don't eat any meat or dairy. I feel really good about eating this way. I don't think anything is hard about it. When my friends ask me why I don't eat meat, I ask them why they eat meat if they like animals. My family eats this way because we don't like eating things that were alive, and to be healthy. I like being vegan because my food doesn't smell bad.

I like to play sports, and if I eat this way it will help me be stronger. I don't get sick very much, and if I do get sick it doesn't last very long. I know when I go on my mission I might have to eat some meat and dairy, but Heavenly Father will help me because I try not to.

*Bradshaw Hirschi is 9 and lives in Coeur d'Alene, Idaho with his parents, three brothers, and one sister. He likes soccer and is crazy about baseball. He enjoys school most of the time, especially PE.*

---

I have not ever had meat in my whole life. I like to be vegan because I don't need to worry about having cancer, heart attacks, stroke, etc. I have never been tempted to eat any thing like meat, cheese, eggs, or anything like that. I have never had any problems with my friends. They all think its cool to be vegan.

A few weeks ago I went to an overnight camp for all the sixth graders. It was three days long so I would be eating the foods that the cooks made. We knew I would need to bring my own food so we got the menu for the three days. Most of the meals I could not have. Like breakfast burritos and nachos. So the night I was going to camp me and my mom went shopping for my food. At camp I could tell the kids in my group were wondering why I was eating differently, so I told them that I was vegan and had to eat different foods. My teachers always made sure I had the right foods. I am glad I went to camp. We had a lot of fun.

By following the Word of Wisdom I am healthier, happier, and more active than others.

We don't have foods like oreos, doughnuts, cookies, chips, etc. I love all those things but we make our own cookies and cakes, and I think they are delicious. Even better than the ones people buy from stores. We even make cookie dough out of chickpeas! My parents love me so much so they keep my body healthy and active by not feeding me meat and dairy and by following the Word of Wisdom.

*Shayne Hirschi is 11 and lives in Coeur d'Alene, Idaho. She loves gymnastics, swimming, and jumping on the trampoline.*

# Teens

I'm in a family that has been vegan for as long as I remember. It is definitely a big part of my life. My family eats this way because we all have some form of lactose intolerance, and my mom believes it is healthier for us to eat vegan—plus meat grosses us out immensely. Sometimes being vegan is really hard because kids at school will bring really yummy looking food from home, and it's really hard for me to say no when they offer some to me.

Whenever people ask why I'm vegan, I say so I can be healthy without exercising. That usually shuts them up.

The Word of Wisdom also helps me when I'm telling my friends why I'm vegan. One of my friends, who was jokingly trying to convince me to un-veganize, told me that in the Word of Wisdom it even says we can eat meat! So I told her, "Yeah, *sparingly* and in times of FAMINE! Are we in a time of famine? I think NOT!"

I find it easier to tell people I'm vegan when the Word of Wisdom backs me up on it. I love being vegan, because I know what I'm eating is good for me, and I don't feel gross after I eat something. I can also really tell a difference when I'm very strict about being vegan. I can exercise longer and harder, and I don't get headaches as much.

One time when I was younger I had a really big operation on my leg. The doctor said it would take me a minimum of six months for my leg bone to heal. At three months, we went to the doctor's for my weekly checkup, and I got some x-rays taken. When we talked with the doctor, we found out my leg had completely healed. My doctor jokingly said, "You must have drunk a lot of milk!" My mom and I just looked at each other and laughed—on the contrary! I know that because I chose to follow the Word of Wisdom my body healed faster, which was huge blessing.

*Liesel Allen is 14. She's an identical twin, loves to swim, and is learning how to rock climb. Liesel lives in Malaysia, where her father works for the US government.*

Almost a year ago, I decided to stop eating meat. I have stomach issues—problems with digestion that run in the family. When I eat meat or diary,

I end up in the bathroom about an hour later. My mother heard about a plant-based diet from her hairdressing clients [Debbie Christofferson and Ilene Christensen], so we decided to go the vegetarian route.

About a year before deciding to go vegetarian, I started to be very interested in health and taking care of my body, so this decision felt like a natural next step. I felt it would help me. Then as we did some research, and I learned what it really means to be vegetarian and what it really means to be vegan, I decided why not go the extra step and be a full-on vegan? So I've been doing that the past year, and it has helped me a lot with my stomach. I don't have stomach issues with food any more, which is a big thing.

I actually like eating different, more healthy foods. I like knowing there are different ways to eat. Probably the thing I like most is finding the things you can eat that you didn't know about before and learning that they actually taste good. People think vegans eat dirt as their main food, but there are all kinds of things vegans eat. I like it.

I'm not hesitant to talk about my diet with others, but I don't shout about being vegan from the rooftop. Friends sometimes ask me, "Why do you like that?" Most kids are not vegetarian, and especially not vegan, and for a guy it is really unusual. I tell them it helps me with my stomach, but that it is not just for my health—I do it because I want to. They don't give me a hard time, but they think it is weird. Whether they like it or not doesn't really impact me.

I'm not tempted by animal foods, but I do miss ice cream. My dad likes to tempt me. He says he is trying to make sure I'm walking the walk. He has learned that I don't cave in no matter how much he tries to get me to eat things I don't eat any more, and he is actually very proud of me for doing what I feel is right and sticking by my decision. He even told me that he looks to me for strength to make some health decisions he has to make. My dad actually does a lot of the shopping and cooking, so my diet has impacted him almost more than me. My 13-year-old sister thinks I'm crazy, but she knows this diet has been good for me.

If I am tempted to eat something not good for me, I just tell myself to not eat it. You have to have good will power. It is not easy. You have to understand it is not easy. You have to stick to it. I feel better when I stick to it. I feel gross when I eat sugar or things that I usually don't eat because of the diet. I can just tell.

When people read the Word of Wisdom, they mostly focus on the drinking and smoking part and then go right to the "run and not be weary" part, but they don't pay attention to the part about eating herbs in season and not eating meat as much and eating meat in times of winter or times of famine. They skip the 7-8 verses about eating healthy. I don't think the Word of Wisdom says "don't eat meat, don't eat dairy," but I think it goes well with being vegan.

Besides helping me to keep healthy, being vegan has helped me be more active. I feel I have more energy when I'm swimming. I also think it helps me have a clear mind, and possibly stay more in tune with the Spirit. I am definitely more in tune with what my body needs. Because I feel so good, I can concentrate more on what is needed during the day.

My mom is very proud of me. She is glad I'm learning to take care of myself now while I'm still living at home. She believes that after I leave home, when I pray about what I should eat and how to fuel my body, the answers will come quicker because I am more in tune with what my body needs.

*Michael Anderson, 16, lives in Logan, Utah and is a sophomore at Logan High, where he is on the Logan High swim team. Michael plays piano and viola. He loves to spend time with friends, compose music, and talk to his lab, Libby.*

## The 20's

While I was growing up, healthy eating was important in my family. My mother had been a vegetarian for most of her married life, so she always insisted on our eating "healthy" food. We were far from vegan (we still consumed dairy), but we hardly ever had meat in our house, except when my dad made his delicious tri-tip steaks. We also had very few processed foods.

Later, both my parents became vegan, and the few animal products still in the house gradually began disappearing. Dairy milk was replaced with soy, almond, or rice milk. Meat was no longer an option, even on special occasions. More emphasis was placed on eating fruits and vegetables. I begrudgingly went along with the plan, seeing there weren't many other food options at home. I loved going to friends' houses or eating out because I could eat all the junk I wanted. I had no appreciation for a healthy diet.

This all changed the day my mom issued me a challenge: "Why don't you just try going completely vegan for a week? You can see how you feel and decide whether to continue."

So I did. I completely stopped eating meat, dairy, and eggs. I also stopped eating any processed foods, including sugar. I was about 16 years old at the time, and I was running distance in track and cross-country. I noticed that when I started eating whole foods my stamina and ability to endure increased.

I was able to recover faster between workouts. I had more energy during school. I just felt clean! And this was only after one week of eating this way ! ! During the next three years, I ate a diet completely untainted by animal products or processed foods. I felt the best I had ever felt in my whole life.

It was difficult at first though, especially socially. Most of my friends could not understand why I would eat this way. I was often asked questions like, "Where do you get your protein (calcium, vitamin B12, etc.)?" or, "If dairy is so bad for my health, then why doesn't my doctor warn me?" At first, I didn't know what to say. All I knew is that I felt better eating this way, and my mom said it was good for me. Being frustrated at how little I really knew about nutrition, I decided to study it out for myself.

Coming to a knowledge of a whole foods diet seems to parallel how I gained a testimony of the gospel. At first I blindly believed because that is how I was raised, and it felt good. But as time went on, I realized I would need to study it out and really find out for myself if it was right. My mom was a great help. She directed me to books like *The China Study* and other credible sources where I could learn more about the science or "why's" of eating this way. Most importantly, she encouraged me to study the Word of Wisdom. I thought I knew everything there was to know about the Word of Wisdom, but I couldn't have been more wrong. As I studied the verses of Section 89 again, my eyes were opened. I found "wisdom and great treasures of knowledge, even hidden treasures" (D&C 89:19). The Word of Wisdom is an inspired nutritional guide for optimum health!

When I was nineteen, I was called to serve a mission in Argentina, the "meat capital of the world." Those who know me asked how I would survive if I had to eat meat for two years. In preparation for a mission, the possibility of having to put my vegan diet on hold had crossed my mind. I decided the Lord would bless me if I did my best to be healthy, while at the same time focusing on the most important task at hand, the salvation of God's children. When we ate with members, or when people offered us food, I would eat a helping of everything. I was very careful not to offend anybody by refusing their food. Although my body was not used to this at first, I found that it worked out. I felt extremely blessed, especially since I was able to eat plenty of fruits and vegetables back at the apartment. My companions and other missionaries noticed this, and some of them started following suit. The "green drinks" I made every morning became famous and spread like wildfire throughout the mission.

During the two years of my mission, I learned a great deal about how eating a whole foods, plant-based diet relates to the gospel. I came to understand that the Word of Wisdom is counsel that I treasure greatly, but it is not the most important part of my life. I realized that things like faith, repentance, obedience to the commandments, and gospel ordinances are the *most* important aspects of the gospel, and therefore merit most of my attention. I also realized, however, how blessed I truly feel to understand how the Lord wants each of us to eat, and that it pleases Him when we take care of our bodies. Needless to say, it was very refreshing to start back up on a vegan diet after returning home.

Since I got back from my mission, I have thrived on this diet. I have noticed its effects in all facets of my life, but mostly in my athletic endeavors. I have competed in several triathlons and distance running competitions, some in which I have placed first and set course records. I love to push the limits of my body and see how much "grit" I really have. You can find me day-in-and-day-out trail-running, biking, and swimming. I owe my success in these sports largely to the way I eat. I feel the Lord's promises in D&C 89 are directed right at me: "And all saints who remember to keep and do these sayings . . . shall run and not be weary, and shall walk and not faint" (D&C 89:18, 20).

*Victor Johnson, 22, lives in Orem, Utah and is attending BYU. He loves being in the outdoors: running, hiking, swimming, cycling, target shooting, and camping. He also enjoys competing in triathlons and long distance races.*

*You can find the stories for Victor's father, Paul Johnson, at the end of chapter 6 and his for mother, Orva Johnson, later in this appendix.*

---

I am 26 years old and have weighed a sprightly 100 pounds since seventh grade. I never gave much thought to what I ate, since candy, French fries and ice cream didn't seem to affect me negatively, at least in the sense that they never added any pounds to my slight figure. And did I ever take advantage of my unbelievably good genes! As a missionary in France, my motto was, "Why buy one pastry when you can buy two?"

During my last year as an undergraduate, I was working with Jane Birch when she made her radical diet change. I was fairly skeptical of all she preached at first and told myself that, though great for her, it probably wasn't for me. After all, eating a handful of carrot sticks and three different kinds of fruit every day meant I was pretty healthy myself . . . right?

A few months later over Christmas break, my husband and I watched the documentary *Forks Over Knives* and discussed Jane's new lifestyle. Almost on a whim, we decided to try it out and be totally dedicated to a whole foods, plant-based lifestyle for the next three months. My husband was studying nutrition, with plans to go to medical school. He was also interested in losing some weight, being healthier in general, and finding relief from his migraine headaches. I remember eating a frozen pizza that day and wondering how I was going to make it for three months without cheese.

After we changed our diet, we immediately felt we had much more energy. It was invigorating to eat a meal and feel totally satisfied but not heavy or gross from ingesting a bunch of grease or meat. My husband's headaches became less frequent. He lost weight. We felt great! For the first time in my life, I was truly more aware of what I was putting into my body and recognizing the effects food had on me. We knew we were eating much healthier, but we also couldn't believe how delicious our meals were! Our food tasted better than it ever had. We even began evangelizing because it affected us so much.

I was afraid before we decided to do this that my husband would want to keep it going longer than three months. I wasn't sure I could do it forever. Admittedly, two years later, we are not 100% whole food, plant-based—we do eat some fish and cheese occasionally, and my sweet tooth sometimes gets its way—but we follow the Word of Wisdom much more than we ever used to. We have thought significantly more about the do's of the Word of Wisdom rather than focusing on the don'ts and calling it good. This decision has been one of the most life changing for us both, and the whole food, plant-based lifestyle is still very much a part of our lives.

*Robyn Rowley, 26, lives in Silver Spring, Maryland. She earned a BS in Psychology and is currently putting her husband, Dallin, through medical school while working as a healthcare transcriptionist. They are expecting their first baby.*

# The 30's

During couple scripture study one night in 2009, my husband and I read and discussed D&C 89. I asked about the significance of the verses that talk about eating meat sparingly, only in times of cold, winter, and famine. I wondered why we never talk about those verses at church, and whether those verses mean eating an essentially vegetarian diet. We didn't come to a satisfactory conclusion, so I spent a night doing research online. I discovered there are Latter-day Saints who are vegetarian and read about how the Word of Wisdom had influenced them as they decided to change their diets. As I learned more, I knew I could no longer eat meat and felt strongly prompted that giving it up was the right thing for me to do.

At that point, my husband and I hadn't been eating meat very much anyway, mostly because I hated touching raw meat and thought it was too expensive. We were pretty healthy eaters since we had given up processed food and refined sugars three years earlier. My husband was supportive of this change to our eating habits. We have a deal: he can buy all the meat he wants as long as he buys it, cooks it, and stays within our grocery budget, which he does a few times a year.

After removing processed food, refined sugars, and meat from our diets, my husband and I both lost a lot of weight and felt a lot healthier. My doctor thought I was lactose-intolerant and had irritable bowel syndrome (IBS), a condition that can actually be made worse by eating whole grains. After removing processed foods and meat from my diet, the IBS symptoms stopped, my tension headaches disappeared, and I no longer consider myself lactose-intolerant.

I used to hate cooking, but giving up processed food, refined sugars, and meat gave me a drive to learn how to cook delicious, healthy meals. I started collecting as many recipes as I could, trying out multiple ones every day so I would have a huge repertoire of healthy meals. I learned to love cooking, and my skills increased the more I did it. We've expanded our eating horizons to include all sorts of things I never ate growing up. I learned to love brown rice, whole wheat pasta, and dozens of fruits, vegetables, and other whole grains. I even learned to love broccoli, my childhood nemesis. In a way, removing meat from my diet forced me to investigate and learn to like new foods—foods that are much healthier for me than the meat they replaced. I now consider myself an adventurous eater, willing to try all sorts of foods I never ate growing up. My husband says I am an amazing cook, and he is impressed with all of the foods he thought he didn't like but now loves. We love this way of eating and would never go back.

In 2012, I picked up a copy of *The China Study* at a used bookstore and flipped through it. Despite having heard so much good press about it, I chose not to buy it. I felt like it was "preaching to the choir" since I already had given up meat, and I felt uncomfortable with the thought of giving up dairy and eggs as well. But I started receiving more promptings after that point about giving up dairy and eggs—sometimes when reading the Word of Wisdom, sometimes when thinking about my diet, and once when reading about a new study that showed that eggs raise your risk of heart disease (which runs in my family). I didn't think it was possible for me to give them up, so I ignored the promptings, but 15 months later, in 2013, I finally listened to the promptings, read *The China Study*, watched *Forks Over Knives*, and decided to stop eating dairy and eggs.

By giving up meat, I experience a greater clarity when I read the Word of Wisdom and other scriptural verses that discuss food and the relationship between man and animals. I have more compassion for animals and a greater understanding of what it means to be a steward over the earth. I know animals have the right to fulfill the measure of their creation and have joy, and they can't do that when they're living in such horrible, unnatural conditions. I am happy I don't contribute to the suffering of animals caused by eating meat, dairy, and eggs, and it gives me peace to know that I can please God by not eating His animals. I am sure I displease God in many things, but I am happy to know I can please Him in this area.

I now have a much greater testimony that the Word of Wisdom was truly given for our day! In a world where contradictory nutritional information abounds, the Word of Wisdom is the standard we should use.

*Christie Cosky, 31, lives in Orem, Utah. She has a BS in Computer Science and works as a software engineer. She loves reading, running, programming, and trying new recipes. She also enjoys hiking, camping, and watching science fiction movies with her husband.*

---

From the time I was thirteen I thought I was fat. I tried every diet imaginable and read every weight-loss book I could get my hands on. I would do anything to be skinny: drink lemonade for ten days, count calories, hire personal trainers. I pled with the Lord to just show me the right way to lose weight. Ironically, I was never more than ten pounds overweight.

About seven years ago, the Lord led me down a different path, a path that changed my focus from outward appearances to true health.

It was then that I was introduced to cancer. No—it wasn't me. But suddenly cancer was "everywhere." A good friend, two neighbors, close family friends and loved ones were all diagnosed within a very short period of time. I was shaken. My prayers changed. *Heavenly Father, is there something I should learn here? Is there something you could teach me—something that would protect my family?*

In July of 2008, an article entitled "Cancer, Nutrition and the Word of Wisdom" jumped right out of the *Ensign* and spoke to my heart: *Charity, you are not following the Word of Wisdom as you ought.* I had just hired my second trainer at the gym and was following an eating plan that included six small meals a day, all including animal protein. As I read the article, I knew I needed to change. But I didn't know how.

Shortly thereafter, I was introduced to Colin Campbell's *The China Study.* Once again my soul was shaken. It felt like truth. It felt like a gift. I was thankful, but I also felt anger: why had I been deceived for so long by our society and our Standard American Diet? I felt lost. I knew I wanted to change, for myself and for my four children, but how? *I'm ready, Father, but I don't know how. I don't know how to do this, and I need your help.*

Enter Dr. Joel Fuhrman. After reading his wonderful book, *Eat to Live,* I was ready to dive into this new world. I read anything I could get my hands on—studying, pondering, searching, and praying. I was filled with fire and became passionate about sharing my new knowledge. I started a business focused on in-home, whole food cooking parties. I became certified as a Plant-based Nutritionist through eCornell. I co-founded the plant-based, family-oriented website www.wholefoodmommies.com and became a "Food for Life" instructor (which is how I met Jane Birch).

The Lord has blessed me every step of the way: with like-minded people who are uplifting and encouraging, with sources of light and knowledge that keep me developing my desire for good health, and with a new perspective on the body I was given. I've learned that my HEALTH is so much more important than how I look. There is a fine line between eating for health and eating for vanity. I sometimes cross that line, but deep down I have peace. My spirit is happy, and I know this way of eating is the best way for my *spirit* to progress and grow. (Had I been one of those "skinny girls," I don't think I would have had a desire to search for this wisdom.)

I do NOT eat perfectly; I never have and probably never will. I have learned not to worry so much about the every-once-in-a-while. Instead I focus on the EVERY DAY: fruits, vegetables and whole grains . . . every day! I find it helpful to concentrate on things I want to include rather than things I exclude.

Eating a plant-based diet can be challenging; anyone who jumps on board should expect opposition. My advice would be to sit back and watch as the adversary (who fully understands the link between your spirit and your physical body) moves in when you do anything to improve your health. Simply see these moments of opposition as clues that you are on track.

Almost every person I know who has TRULY desired to understand the BEST way to care for our bodies has been led to this path. I know the

Word of Wisdom was written for our day. The Lord knew the confusion we would face, and He knew the "conspiring men" who would work to deceive us. He loves us and desires to bless us. He gave us a guide—an instruction manual for our bodies. He knows our bodies are conduits to the spiritual realm. The words He gave us are instructions on how to become closer to Him, how to connect better with Him, and how to receive further light and knowledge (through those glorious "hidden treasures"). As I changed what I put into my body, I could feel my spirit changing too. Growing. Expanding. Seeking more light. I gained a clarity of mind that quickly leaves when I don't pay heed to what I eat—brain fog is the first symptom when I indulge in things I know I shouldn't eat.

I am so grateful for the things the Lord has allowed me to learn. I feel so blessed to live on this earth that provides everything I need to flourish. I am thankful for the wisdom and courage of others who continue to share these wonderful truths with the world.

*Charity Lighten is mother of four and lives in Riverton, Utah. Born in Canada, she met her husband at BYU where she graduated in Accounting. She is currently serving in her very first call with the Young Women as the Stake Young Women's President. She loves to cook, exercise, and travel.*

# The 40's

When my husband's cholesterol crept above 200, his doctor cautioned him to take better care of himself, so we both started working to lose weight. After losing 10 lbs, he had his cholesterol checked again. It was still 204.

A few weeks later, I happened to sit next to Jane Birch at a meeting. When I commented on how lean she was looking, she promptly introduced me to whole food, plant-based eating. After reading *The China Study* at her recommendation, I talked my husband into trying the diet with me. Six weeks later, we were both down about 15 lbs He got his cholesterol checked again. It was 131. Amazing!

His cholesterol came down so fast and easily, though, I guess we weren't really convinced of the importance of continuing to eat that way. Over the next several months we gradually went back to old patterns, especially during the holidays, and his cholesterol began creeping right back up. We realized that in order to avoid heart disease, we'd have to get the cholesterol down and keep it down.

My cholesterol has never been considered high, although it did climb from the 120s to the 170s over the past couple of decades of fast-food living. More important to me, though, was the way I was feeling overall. I used to feel smart, but now my mind felt foggy, and it was hard to remember things and to come up with creative ideas. My stomach hurt every day. I was always tired and couldn't sit still for more than about 30 minutes without falling asleep. I started waking up with nagging headaches that would last most of the day. Joints and muscles hurt randomly for no good reason. After work I felt worn out with no energy left for anything else.

We decided to make a new beginning with the whole food, plant-based lifestyle, and this time stick with it. I knew the hardest part would be the first few days when my body craved the kind of junk it had grown used to: sugar, fat, salt, and, for me, constant munching. After the first few days (which were pretty rough), the cravings went away, and I started feeling really good. We weren't hungry—we ate huge portions of vegetables, fruits, and greens at every meal. After the first week or so, those foods started to taste delicious. Flavors seemed stronger. Sweetened foods became less appealing than before because it seemed like the sugar was just covering the real flavors. I've found some wonderful recipes, and it's been so much fun trying them out. I now have no headaches, no stomach pains, and enough energy left to go do something fun after work each day.

The whole food, plant-based way of eating isn't a "diet" in the short-term sense of the word. It's a lifestyle. You have to approach it that way to be successful. I've tried diets before, trying to combat the slower metabolism that arrived with middle age. I'm embarrassed to admit how many: Atkins, cabbage soup, weight loss shakes, SunChips and Diet Coke (I invented that one), McDonalds for breakfast and then little else all day long (also my invention). Some of them made me lose weight, for a little while. None of them made me feel good. While I was eating that way, I knew I was violating the advice given in the Word of Wisdom, but I always told myself I would only do it for a little while until I lost the weight. It sounds so foolish, but I'm sure I'm not the only one who tells myself things like that.

I am thrilled to see how perfectly this diet fits with the Word of Wisdom. Doctors and scientists who have no connection to the LDS Church are now giving people the same advice God gave us through Joseph Smith nearly two centuries ago. That, together with the way I feel now, has me firmly convinced that a whole food, plant-based lifestyle is the way to live a healthy and productive life, with enough energy to accomplish everything I want to do while enjoying every day along the way. I feel so good!

*Laura C. Bridgewater, PhD, 46, lives in Provo, Utah and is a professor in the Department of Microbiology and Molecular Biology at Brigham Young University. She and her husband have four adult children. She enjoys bicycling, snow skiing, water skiing, cooking, reading, and being in the mountains.*

My journey to a plant-based diet began soon after my diagnosis with prostate cancer. However, to begin fully, I should probably start earlier. My grandmother passed away from cancer, after being terrified of the big 'C' from youth. My mother passed away from lung cancer; then a few years later, my wife's only sister developed breast cancer. She ended up having a mastectomy, followed by chemotherapy and radiation.

I had been called as bishop of a very busy ward in New Zealand. One of my first challenges was dealing with a single sister with two teenage children who had breast cancer, but refused to get treatment or let me tell anyone. The week my sister-in-law finished her radiation treatment, our 15-year-old daughter developed what was thought to be a form of leukemia. We were devastated. It was a harrowing time but through a ward fast and miracles, her life was spared.

In December 2008, a close friend, who was more like an older brother, was diagnosed with aggressive prostate cancer. His PSA reading was 300 (4 or below is considered normal). I thought prostate cancer was an older man's disease, but he was in his late 50's—at the time I was 43 years old.

One day the following April (2009), as I was driving past our local chapel, the Spirit whispered to me, "Get a PSA test." Because it was such a strong prompting, I didn't delay. Our GP [general practitioner] is a neighbor, friend, and LDS. On arriving at his office, I suddenly felt very silly asking for a PSA test, but I plucked up the courage to tell him why I was there. When he heard I had no symptoms, he told me, "You don't even start getting tested until you are 50. You are too young." But I felt a strong prompting to push for the test and almost demanded one. He replied, "If it makes you sleep better tonight, have a test, but I can guarantee you will be fine."

To make a long story short, I wasn't fine. Many tests later, I had a confirmed diagnosis of prostate cancer. The first person I called was my wife, who was upset, but we discussed that things would be okay, and that I needed to tell our children that night. So at Family Home Evening I had to sit the four children down to explain that I had cancer.

I spent the next day trying to think my way through the situation, but the more I thought the more confused I became. That night I ended up at the New Zealand Temple, where I pled with the Lord, "I have a family who has been through so much, Father. I have a ward that needs me, and a job that I'm finding a challenge." Suddenly, I remembered my patriarchal blessing, which promised me two gifts (1) the ability to solve my own problems and (2) the gift of discernment to choose wisely. I said to the Lord, "I have these gifts. I need to use them. PLEASE help me."

I stared down at my lap, and the scriptures I was holding opened to Section 89. My heart started racing, like it does when you feel the prompting to bear your testimony, and I felt compelled to read the passage. I immediately had two thoughts: (1) this could be a coincidence . . . after all, I knew everything there was about the Word of Wisdom (I had even taught a fireside on it!); or (2) it was the Lord trying to tell me something. I chose there and then to believe the Lord wanted me to read this. I felt He was telling me, "This is an answer to the problem. Read it and you can solve it."

I read the verses in front of me. When I came to verse 13, my heart started racing: "*And it is pleasing unto me that they should not be used*"! At this stage I was a meat eater. I loved ice cream and ate a typical Western diet. I weighed around 95 kg (209 lbs), which at 179 cm (5'10") seemed to be okay. However I instantly felt the answer I was seeking was somehow related to food. Could food cause cancer?

I went home that night and jumped on the Internet and soon started to find page after page ("hidden treasures") that associated increased animal protein intake with cancer. I was pretty gobsmacked! Could this be true? I was VERY skeptical and kept trying to find evidence to the contrary. Yes, there was conflicting evidence, but it was also accompanied by further evidence of animal protein causing not just cancer but heart disease too. I absolutely didn't want to believe it, but the next day I cut down a little on the meat I was eating.

At my next appointment with the specialist I asked him outright, "Could my cancer be related to food?" The specialist was a very good man, who I liked, but he said, "No, not at all, eat what you like."

I came away feeling very confused but decided the prompting I had received was just too strong to ignore, so that day I cut almost all animal protein out of my diet. My wife was upset, as were our children. I immediately started losing weight. People in the ward were worried. They thought my weight loss was due to the cancer, when in fact it was the diet.

Because it was not easy, I was ready to give up on my new diet. Then one morning I woke up and something was different. I felt "high." I felt clear. It hit me: I'd had a really good night's sleep as my nose was not blocked at all. My nose had been consistently blocked from around age 17—around the same time I started my first job, had full access to dairy, and soon developed a taste for it. My healing continued . . . a few weeks later a painful shoulder condition which had plagued me for years suddenly disappeared. On the day of my surgery in September I was amazed to find I had lost around 22 kg (48.5 lbs) in a few months.

But after a four-to-five-hour major surgery, I just wanted my life to be like it was before, so I had a chicken sandwich! So, the "absolutely no meat-eating phase" didn't last, but despite this I still couldn't deny the promptings I had received. For the next few months I struggled on a mostly plant-based diet, ignoring the Internet, as I was just so confused and conflicted with all of the information available. I did however feel really well for the most part, and my energy levels increased dramatically. My family members were unhappy with me and were encouraging me to eat more meat.

One weekend, while on a hike, someone mentioned that he'd heard I was a wannabe vegan. I explained how I was feeling and that the information on the Internet was confusing and contradictory. He said I should read two books. One of them was called *The China Study*. I parked the information in the back of my mind. That week, in an attempt to find more support for a vegetarian diet, I went to a Seventh-day Adventist recipe class. That first night the presenter said we should all read a very important book: *The China Study*. Once again, I thought it was strange, but just parked it away in my mind.

A couple of months later, in April 2010, my job took me to Omaha, Nebraska for ten days. While I was there, my diet well and truly slipped. The first night there was a gift basket left on my bed, with chocolate and chips. The company café offered meat galore. I went to an employee's home for dinner and had a piece of rare steak. I just wanted to feel "normal." Why couldn't I eat meat? Underneath it all I still felt that the promptings I'd had were right, but I was struggling to reconcile them with the life I wanted.

On the day I flew back to New Zealand, I was at the LA airport where I ended up walking into a small bookshop and instantly remembered the book that had been mentioned. A small Hispanic lady was putting books away when I asked her if she had heard of *The China Study*. She literally squealed and explained she'd just had a copy in her hand. Then, without moving, she turned and pulled a copy off the shelf behind her. I took it as another sign and bought it!

I found a quiet place and bowed my head in prayer. I told Heavenly Father I had bought a book and asked if I could have wisdom to discern the truth out of it. Then, as I read, I felt that the puzzle pieces of information stored in my brain were like a Rubik's Cube that had just come together! I was engrossed. I felt, and still feel, the book contained truth. It was one of the many "hidden treasures" I would subsequently find. At that point my whole attitude changed, and I went totally plant-based.

My energy and clarity increased dramatically, and my reasons for going plant-based changed too. Suddenly I was eating plant-based, not only for my health, but for other sentient beings—as well as the environment. Within two months of my reading *The China Study*, my wife, who had been very skeptical, also read it. She became plant-based and experienced even greater health benefits than I.

I have changed so much over the past three plus years. My perspective has changed. I love life. I meditate, do Bikram yoga, and run barefoot (previously I couldn't run due to knee pain). I have even started a blog. My wife has joined me on this journey, which has been awesome—we've even held classes together at church meetings about this topic.

It hasn't always been easy and most days we face questions from people—some who are genuinely curious and some who just want to rubbish a plant-based diet. We just keep on going. With the health benefits we've experienced, we don't need to listen to any other perspectives—we just trust the spirit. Now, more and more people who had initially been skeptical are asking questions, with several starting the transition to a plant-based diet.

Yes, of course illness could strike again, but now our lives are all about quality, not quantity. I want to feel how I feel now. I feel so alive. I feel great. This is how I think everyone should feel and how Heavenly Father wants each of us to feel.

I believe in the blessings of the Word of Wisdom—we are still uncovering treasures of hidden knowledge, and I'm certainly running without being weary . . . in fact I'm training for my first half marathon!

*Kevin Tunstall, 48, lives in Hamilton, New Zealand. He is married to Gay-lynn, and they have four children, three daughters and one son. Kevin works in the finance industry. Apart from taking a keen interest in nutrition, Kevin also enjoys Bikram yoga and barefoot running.*

# The 50's

My journey to a whole food, plant-based diet has been wonderful! I have felt guided, inspired, and so blessed to gradually have the truth revealed to me about how I should eat.

I grew up in a family that used whole grains and tried to avoid refined sugar. I tried to continue with these values when I had my own family. Almost 30 years ago I was persuaded to cut dairy milk out of my diet because our sixth daughter had terrible colic. Cutting the dairy from my diet helped her so much—I was very motivated. By the time I was done nursing her, I no longer missed the dairy.

About that same time, I made a new friend, Julene Humes, who became a mentor to me. Julene was way ahead of me in her understanding of nutrition. She helped me *thoroughly comprehend* the downside of animal foods. I took things a step at a time: first no dairy, then no meat, and finally no eggs. I still used milk and eggs to bake for my family but ate very little of them myself. This new knowledge felt so right, and I knew I was being guided in the changes I was making. I gained a rich appreciation for the verses of the Word of Wisdom that go beyond "temple worthiness."

Then my husband, Paul, developed pre-diabetes and some other health problems about ten years ago. I was discussing his health issues with a friend and physical therapist, Rogan Taylor, who took the opportunity to introduce me to *The China Study*. I read it and urged Paul to try a 100% vegan diet as an experiment. After three months on a strict whole food, plant-based diet he was basically cured. His blood sugar numbers were completely normal. He saw this as good and bad news: good that he didn't have diabetes—bad that he knew he should cut out all animal foods. (Paul later joked with Rogan that it was his fault he could no longer eat meat.) Since then we have been pretty strict about following a plant-based diet in our home. I do not feel deprived because I really love the foods we eat.

Over the years I have become convinced that eating a whole food, plant-based diet is the best for me. I find real joy in seeing our seven married children eating this way. Our 22-year-old son, Victor, also loves to eat healthy food. He is very athletic and active and feels a whole food, plant-based diet helps him perform his best. Our youngest son, a senior in high school, eats what I fix at home but is happy to eat meat, cheese, and junk with his friends. I think he believes our food is healthier but is not ready to go 100% yet.

I am told in my patriarchal blessing that I should always remember the example I can be through the Word of Wisdom. I used to be confused about what that meant. Most of my friends are LDS and already believe in the Word of Wisdom. Finding new hidden treasures of knowledge about nutrition has become a delightful hobby of mine. I LOVE the Word of Wisdom and feel it was given for our time, even more than when it was revealed to the Prophet Joseph. It is a standard by which to measure all the worldly theories about diet. I appreciate our amazing bodies and am so grateful we have been given revelation on how to take care of them.

*Orva Johnson, 57, lives in Orem, Utah. She and her husband Paul have nine children and will have 30 grandchildren by the end of the year. She loves her family and enjoys reading, sewing, and being outdoors. She does Bikram yoga for fun and to keep in shape. Orva and her daughters share their favorite WFPB recipes with each other and friends, known and unknown, on their website GreenerEating.com.*

*Orva Johnson is an example of the impact one dedicated mother can have on the health and habits of an entire family. After deciding to eat plant-based herself, nearly her entire family has converted through her example. But each child, and now each grandchild, has had to "gain their own testimony" of the value of a whole food, plant-based diet.*

*You can find the story of Orva's husband, Paul, at the conclusion of chapter 6. Orva's sister, Elna Clark, is featured in the next story. A few of Orva's grandchildren (Sally, Elaine, Mariah, Bradshaw, Shayne, and Liesel) and her son, Victor, were featured earlier in this appendix. Several of her daughters have also written their stories, and they are featured on the website, discoveringthewordofwisdom.com.*

Twenty-five years ago I had colon cancer and had to have part of my colon removed. There were complications following my surgery, and digestion became more and more difficult. The doctors could do very little to help, and I did nothing to change my diet at that time.

About five years ago I started getting some arthritis-like symptoms. Rheumatologists were not certain what to call what I had, but at its worst I couldn't get out of bed or even hold my hand up to my ear to hold the phone. For a few years I was on Prednisone, but that obviously was not a good permanent solution.

My sister, Orva Johnson, suggested I give up ALL animal foods. I had already eliminated all dairy (except for butter) from my diet several years earlier because I found it wreaked havoc on my digestive system. Also, I ate VERY little meat, maybe a half cup per week. Butter was my weakness. In a way I thought I was so close to being vegan already, how much difference could the extra small changes make? But I knew I needed to get off Prednisone, and the pain of the arthritis was debilitating.

So, I did it. I gave up all animal foods and started living a whole food, plant-based lifestyle. Within weeks, I had gone off the Prednisone and was no longer in any pain. I am very grateful. Since then, reading and hearing the things I do about a whole food, plant-based diet, I would not switch back even if I had no arthritis to deal with.

I definitely see the Word of Wisdom differently now. In a way, I can't figure out how I ever justified my eating practices. In our day and age, I don't see when our circumstances would qualify as "times of winter, or of cold, or famine." With food available at all times in stores, we don't live the life our ancestors did. My restoration to health without pain is a blessing, which I associate with living the Word of Wisdom.

*Elna Clark, 58, lives in Fairfield, California. She and her husband have six children and eight grandchildren. She is a pianist and enjoys quilting and reading.*

# The 60's

Originally, I didn't give much thought to the Word of Wisdom, except to follow the directions needed to be baptized in my early twenties (1972) and obtain a temple recommend a year later. That changed in 2011, when I became a vegan. It all began when I watched a video posted on Facebook called "Best Speech You Will Ever Hear" by Gary Yourofsky, an American animal rights activist. His presentation was about the atrocities that we humans do and allow to happen to animals, for unnecessary food and entertainment. That very day, out of compassion for animals, I became a vegan. My youngest daughter was very happy to join me in this new way of living, and my husband, without even looking at the information, was okay about it too.

We live in Temple View, Hamilton, New Zealand in a community where the population is about 97% Latter-day Saint, with very few less active. For the next two years, as far as I knew, we were the only vegans here. There were five wards in Temple View at the time, and only later did I discover that one of the ward bishops, Kevin Tunstall, had become vegan two years earlier than us, and his wife and daughter had joined him.

Since becoming a vegan, I've spent my time learning everything I can, from recipes, to animal rights, to health issues. We began by eating the same meals as before, minus the animal products. As I discovered the huge amount of information about the health benefits of a whole food, plant-based vegan diet, we were further supported in our determination to be permanently vegan and progressed to using whole foods only, no refined and very little processed foods. I had always had a sweet tooth, and I loved to bake desserts and bread products of all kinds, using lots of butter and cream. I applied myself to switching over to the vegan whole food versions of my favorite foods and in the process discovered an appreciation of fruits and vegetables, nuts and seeds, whole grains, plant milks, cold-pressed coconut oil, etc. These foods made us feel so much healthier that my desire to prepare sugary and fatty foods dissipated, much to the relief of my daughter, who is highly motivated to maintain good health. I do still sometimes indulge in less-ideal vegan foods when I'm at an activity or have allowed myself to get hungry, but I am making better choices as time goes by.

I have also become more confident in the ability of my body to protect and even heal itself as it is cleared of all toxins and is provided with natural, nutritious food to maintain all its physiological systems. With this awareness in mind, I made a long list of every single health issue I had and have ticked many of them off since going vegan.

As part of the whole process, I studied all I could about the Word of Wisdom in the scriptures and realized that there was more to the Lord's direction than I had understood over the years. This has helped me in conversations with members of the Church who ask me why we are doing this. I also read all the writings available from our Latter-day prophets and other leaders regarding animals and the Word of Wisdom. I found that almost all of the Latter-day prophets have spoken on these matters.

Through temple attendance, I became more aware that the Lord teaches that all beings are created to fulfill the measure of their creation and have joy therein. How my heart breaks when I consider the plight of animals! It is springtime now, and in the nearby farms I hear the continual grievous bellows of the cows; their calves have been taken from them, and their little boys put to death so humans can have their mother's milk. Each Autumn I cringe when I hear the duck hunters shooting the life-mates of the ducks and swans nearby. At the "free range" egg farm the hens are isolated and punished when they become clucky and desire to sit on their eggs to produce their own chicks. The animals cannot fulfill the measure of their creation; the joy for them is replaced with misery at our hands.

The truths I have learned have allowed me to became a missionary to my, now, dear Facebook friend Carl (who posted the video mentioned above). This year (2013) Carl posted a few inquiries about religion as part of his search for God. He wanted to know what different Church founders and leaders have had to say on the subject of animals in relation to humans. I have been able to share with him a great deal of information, and he responded that it was way more than any other religion.

As a great proponent of health, my husband's number one motivation for veganism is connected to the promises from the Lord in the Word of Wisdom, D&C 89:18–21, that through our obedience we shall receive health, renewal, strength, wisdom, knowledge, treasures, and safety. We believe we can obtain these promises by adhering to the entire Word of Wisdom, not just a part of it.

*Christine Bradley, 64, lives a few minutes walk from the Hamilton, New Zealand Temple and the adjoining Visitors Center, where she enjoys taking non-members as part of her member-missionary efforts. She had been a home-schooling mother for 13 years and is now the Church Stake Centre Coordinating Librarian.*

*You can find Kevin Tunstall's story earlier in this appendix.*

--------

Our nutrition quest began many years ago, long before we became converts to the LDS church. Ellen and I met in 1970 in Boston, Mass., while I was in graduate school at Tufts University. Ellen was working for American Airlines and was traveling all over the world. Eventually, I followed my doctoral advisor and relocated to the University of Oklahoma in Norman. I began to frequent a vegetarian restaurant in Norman, and it changed my course, planting a desire in me to eliminate meat from my diet completely. Meanwhile, Ellen decided to take a year off and move to Telluride, Colorado. She soon befriended neighbors who were vegetarians. She decided that not only did it make sense intellectually, but she also felt compelled to make the change. Up to this point, neither of us had been exposed to anything other than the Standard American Diet. So, nearly 900 miles apart, independently, we both decided to become vegetarians. That was an interesting telephone call.

Ellen moved to Norman, and we married in 1977. At this point I was doing postdoctoral research in chemistry. We began to do extensive research on the subject of nutrition and natural healing. We enjoyed a huge garden from which we primarily ate. We were so interested in what we were learning that I decided to apply to a Naturopathic Medical School in California, and off we went. It was an amazing program and exposed both of us to every modality of natural and alternative healing. In 1980, we had our first child, Shanam. At this point we were primarily eating a plant-based diet, with goat milk products from a nearby farm.

After two years of study in California, I received a strong impression that I should apply to medical school. That decision brought us back to the University of Oklahoma to pursue a medical degree. This was a major shift from a holistic view of healing to a pharmaceutical-based medical approach. I came to realize that my gift was in working with the chronically mentally ill and took the direction of psychiatry. I have since discovered that a healthy diet and lifestyle can make a big difference in mental wellness, as well as physical well being, and there is a growing body of research to substantiate this. I have occasionally had the opportunity to lecture on nutrition and mental wellness to other physicians.

Our daughter, Elana, was born in Norman in 1987. Both our children were raised with organic, fresh foods and have been extremely healthy. They have never had a concerning illness and only one brief earache between them. They still live this way and are both great examples of mental, spiritual, and physical wellness.

In 1999, we moved to the Berkshire Mountains in Massachusetts and met a couple who were from The Church of Jesus Christ of Latter-day Saints. Together Ellen and I had researched many religions for over 25 years. We were amazed to finally find the restored gospel and were soon baptized. We were so excited when we read D&C 89. We had found our people! The Lord gave us a revelation concerning a healthy lifestyle with beautiful promises for our obedience! As far as the promises go, Ellen likes to say, "I would eat grass for the promises in the Word of Wisdom!" We were shocked and dismayed when we went to our first church function and pork was being served. What? Still, to this day, we are saddened by meat being served at church functions. We always eat before we go.

Our son's wife, Bethany, has embraced the Word of Wisdom lifestyle to the point of becoming a health coach and is making a great positive impact in her community and beyond. She has a Facebook site where she and her clients and friends post recipes and helpful information. They have two children (so far) and are raising them with a primarily plant-based diet and fresh foods from the garden. When Bethany and Shanam teach together, he says, "My parents are evidence of the results of a healthy diet and lifestyle. I want to be able to be as active and healthy as they are when I am their age. My father is still able to hike 14,000 foot mountains with me, and they both love to hike, ski, snowshoe, garden, and play with their grandchildren. When I look around at others their age, and even those much younger, I am shocked at how unhealthy and out of shape people are. The choice to make is obvious!"

*Tim (67) and Ellen (64) McGaughy live in American Fork, Utah. Ellen is an avid gardener, creative food artist, and family history consultant. Tim received his BS and PhD in chemistry, studied naturopathic medicine, then went to medical school and is a practicing psychiatrist. Tim and Ellen love hiking the local mountains. They have two children and two grandchildren.*

# The 70's

The "moment" came as I was reading the third chapter of *The China Study* by Colin Campbell. I had been in physical therapy for a couple of months when my PT, Rogan Taylor, asked me about my diet. I proudly told him how healthy I ate: not much red meat with a helping of carbohydrates and veggies. He asked if I would be willing to read a book about nutrition and health. I said, "Yes," and he proceeded to leave the room and return with *The China Study*. I asked him if this book was about not eating meat and if he was a vegetarian. He answered affirmatively and testified that the book was based on many years of scientific research that supported diet as the source of health. Since he had been both a bishop and a member of a stake high council, I jokingly told him I did not know they called vegetarians, let alone vegans, to those positions! He laughed and said his wife, a Relief Society president, and all five of their children were vegans. Needless to say, I was impressed.

I had lost my mother the year before due to a litany of diseases: heart disease, diabetes, lung cancer, and lastly a stroke. I had often said I wanted to avoid such a painful and difficult return to our eternal home. Over time, Rogan and I had talked about life and death, loss and pain, tragedy and courage. His spirit of kindness and understanding touched me and created in me a foundation of respect and trust in this wonderful man. So it was that I left his office carrying the book in anticipation of finding the magical power in its pages that could possibly change my perspective.

The "moment" of my awakening to the Word of Wisdom came as if a switch were turned off in my mind that controlled the desire for any animal products. It was both a spiritual and physiological experience, both exhilarating and repulsing. In that moment, my mind and body recoiled at the thought of ingesting animal foods. This was amazing, since I had eaten animal foods my entire life, and now, at the age of 63, everything I believed about a healthy diet was instantly changed. In that same moment, I felt elated to *know* Joseph Smith, Jr. was a true prophet, for only a man of God could have been given this knowledge. I was filled with the witness of the Holy Ghost that the things I was reading were true, and the Word of Wisdom revealed by our Heavenly Father to Joseph was for our physical and spiritual well being.

Tears filled my eyes, and I felt as if I had always known this is the way to be. For years I had felt a deep connection to all creation—every living creature is a gift and is sacred. Somewhere deep inside I wanted to give up eating animals because they were precious and God's creations. I felt whole in that moment, as if I had come home. I was free.

In the seven years since this great revelation occurred, so many blessings have come to pass. A few months after making the decision to not eat animal products, my husband read *The China Study* and came to the conclusion that eating animal foods was not good for his health either. The health benefits have been enormous. After ten years of taking blood pressure medication, he no longer needs it. His cholesterol was 170 and is now 110. He is very healthy at 78 years old. I had suffered from Irritable Bowel Syndrome (IBS) for years and after just a few months of changing my eating habits, I was almost completely free from the symptoms. My cholesterol dropped from 180 to 152. I am 70 years old and take no medications. I can still teach part time at the university. I cannot believe how good it feels to have so much energy. My "moment of truth" has literally changed every fiber of my being and endowed my spirit with a renewed sense of awe for all God's creatures.

*Sandra Cherry is 70 years young and lives in Woodland Hills, Utah. She earned an MS in Psychology and is adjunct faculty at BYU. Her research is in near-death experiences, and she has served for 18 years on the board of the International Association of Near Death Studies-SLC. She and her husband enjoy their ten grandchildren.*

# The 80's

My daughter, Jane Birch, introduced me to her new whole food, plant-based diet in 2011, a few months before I turned 80 years old. Many years before this, I had changed my diet and lost over 70 pounds to get off medication for Type II diabetes. I thought I was eating a healthy diet, and I was exercising regularly. But as I learned about this new diet, I could see the reason in it. This was confirmed the more I studied the Word of Wisdom and realized this diet matches more perfectly the advice given by the Lord. I felt it would improve my chances of avoiding medical problems as I continue to age, so I started to change my diet, with help from my dear daughter.

I've been very happy with the results. Since starting this diet, I've been able to drop all of the medications I was taking, including ones for high blood pressure and cholesterol. I lost an additional 10 pounds, so I'm back to what I weighed in my early twenties! I never get sick: no colds, no headaches. I have plenty of energy for rigorous exercise, and because I'm never sick, I never miss my daily workout: 50 minutes on the arm and leg elliptical at the local rec center. Instead of feeling fatigued when I'm done, I feel energetic!

I've tried to share my newly found appreciation for the Word of Wisdom with my High Priest's group. Judging from the weight of some of them, those particular brethren of mine appear to be in great need of these words of wisdom, but don't appear ready to put into action these sterling truths. They seem to be content with eating what they like to eat no matter what it may be doing to them!

For me, I really enjoy eating grains, beans, potatoes, leafy green foods, and fruit. I am very grateful the Lord blessed each of us with the entire Section 89 of the D&C. He really knows what's best for His children and even His animals, birds, and fish here on earth, and I want to show respect to Him for His love for me by following His counsel fully.

*Neil Birch, 81, lives in Murray, Utah. He earned a Master of Social Work and retired after 29 years with LDS Family Services. Before that he served for five years as an LDS Indian Seminary coordinator. He is the father of nine (Jane is his oldest) and has 22 grandchildren. He enjoys publishing a weekly LDS blog and working out daily at the gym.*

# Appendix 2

# Why Start Now?

I find many people are immediately attracted to a whole food, plant-based diet, but they are often not motivated to make an immediate, radical change in how they eat. The switch does take effort, and there is no guarantee it will be worth it. If you died in a freak accident a month after changing your diet, it will have been a waste of time. In addition, you may be one of the lucky ones who lives a very long life and never gets a chronic illness. But I'm going to predict that at least 99 percent of the people who make the switch will live long enough to say it was one of the best decisions they ever made.

Of course, many people feel pretty good about their health and aren't worried about imminent disease. They may think this change is too radical, given their current situation, and figure they can always revisit that decision in the future. I can see some logic in this line of thinking, but I can also see some serious pitfalls. In this appendix I'd like to present a few compelling reasons to consider starting this diet now. In Appendix Four I'll present some compelling reasons for going 100 percent.

If you are not ill and you love your food, why consider changing your diet now? When I told a friend this diet could prevent heart attacks, she replied, "I'd love to die of a heart attack!" What she meant was that when it is her time to go, a sudden massive heart attack sounds like a relatively quick and painless way. And it is true that for 25 percent of the cases, sudden death is the first and only sign of heart disease.

Fortunately, 75 percent of people survive a heart attack. But how fun is it to live with chronic heart disease? Some will need bypass surgery, a procedure where they take a vein out of your leg, open your chest, and insert the vein into your heart, turning it into an artery. Other survivors will deal with additional surgery, experience frequent chest pains that limit their mobility, suffer the side effects of multiple drugs, and/or live in fear of various body parts shutting down.

For some people, their diet will not lead to a heart attack, but they might have a stroke, which (if it does not kill them) can affect them not just physically but also mentally and emotionally. Many stroke victims are left with permanent neurological damage affecting their ability to perform even the most basic mental and physical tasks. Stroke is the leading cause of disability in the US. Approximately 75 percent of survivors are so disabled they cannot be employed to full capacity. Stroke victims can spend years relearning how to walk, talk, and take care of themselves.

The number of people affected by these disorders is not trivial. According to the Center for Disease Control (CDC), heart disease is the number one killer in America. Strokes are the third leading cause of death. What is number two? Cancer. And while cancer can be caused by many factors, a leading factor for both the cause of cancer and the rate of its progression is again, diet. I don't think I need to tell you what it must be like to be diagnosed with cancer or to go through treatment. How much better would it be just to start eating better now?

So, diet is intimately related to the top three chronic illnesses in America: heart disease, cancer, and strokes. What are the chances you'll be affected by one of these three? The fact is, unless you are on a radically heart-healthy diet, you already have the arterial disease that leads to heart attack and stroke. If you eat the Standard American Diet, fatty streaks begin developing in your arteries when you are a child. Seventeen percent of teenagers eating a Western diet already have plaques from atherosclerosis (see www.webmd. com/heart-disease/features/atherosclerosis-your-arteries-age-by-age). Even relatively healthy-looking people in their 30's and 40's are beginning to experience heart-related problems. The older you are, the worse your arteries are.

Not only can you *reduce* your chance of having heart disease and most types of strokes through diet, you can virtually *eliminate* it because these two chronic illnesses are almost totally diet related, and therefore are nearly 100 percent preventable. Cancer is also highly related to diet and lifestyle and you can drastically reduce your chance of dying from cancer by changing your diet. Of course, there are many other illnesses you can largely prevent or halt through a radical change in diet, including diabetes, hypertension, kidney stones, kidney disease, osteoporosis, arthritis, and many others.

Beyond avoiding many chronic illnesses, by changing your diet now, you'll enjoy better health for the rest of your life. You'll feel better. You'll lose all the weight you need to lose and keep it off for the rest of your life. You'll look better. You'll have more energy. You won't get sick as often. You'll potentially save thousands of medical dollars over the course of your lifetime. You won't experience some of the constant health issues that may not be life threatening but are very uncomfortable and keep you from operating at your peak. If you aren't convinced yet, here are additional rationales for why you may want to start now, rather than wait until you actually have a chronic illness:

*Prevention is easier than treatment.* Disease is easier to prevent than to manage. Why wait until serious illness strikes? Just think how you feel every time you are seriously ill. When I am sick I always think to myself, "Almost no sacrifice would have been too much to avoid feeling this terrible!" When you are tempted to eat food that is not good for your body, picture yourself in the future with chronic illness. At that time, with all the worry, medical bills, loss of independence, and pain, will you be saying, "Sure I'm suffering now, but those donuts, that cheesecake, all that chicken and beef and processed foods were sure worth it!"?

*Give yourself the chance of achieving optimal health.* By starting now, you'll have a better chance of reaching and maintaining optimal health. If you wait too long, this may never be an option for you.

*Don't be complacent—many debilitating illnesses take years to develop.* This is from an online blogger, the Healthy Librarian: "*Why Am I Following This Diet If I Don't Have Heart Disease?* Because my parents were very sick for many years & I'd prefer to not be. I don't want to end up in a wheelchair, unable to walk, unable to talk, incontinent, unable to feed myself, or recognize my loved ones. Heart disease, strokes, vascular dementia, diabetes, Alzheimer's, and even some cancers can take years to develop. Why wait until it's too late to do something about them?"

*Poor habits lead to poor quality of life.* The following advice is from *30 Lessons for Living: Tried and True Advice from the Wisest Americans.* This is not a book about diet, just advice from some of our oldest citizens—those who have lived long enough to know better: "Act now like you will need your body for a hundred years. Stop using 'I don't care how long I live' as

an excuse for bad health habits. Behaviors like smoking, poor eating habits, and inactivity are less likely to kill you than to sentence you to years
or decades of chronic disease. Think walkers, wheelchairs, nursing homes,
incontinence, dementia, oxygen, social isolation, and years of dependence."

*No one who eats poorly escapes in the end.* Dr. Caldwell Esselstyn answered the question, "Why should I change? My health is excellent," by
stating, "No one escapes in the end—eventually the traditional Western
diet guarantees some form of disease in all of us. While it may not be
heart disease at the moment, eventually it will be hypertension, diabetes,
stroke, obesity, gall stones, diverticulitis, rheumatoid arthritis, lupus, multiple sclerosis, or a greater likelihood of breast, prostate, colon, ovarian
and uterine cancers. Even erectile dysfunction and dementia. The world
famous Framingham Heart Study, now approaching its 60th year, looked
at 1,000 people at age 50 who had normal blood pressure. They looked at
the same group at age 70, and 90 percent now had high blood pressure.
But there is something you can do now to stop the cascading events that
occur in the body and lead to disease. You can change your diet and begin
safeguarding your health for the future."

*It is harder to change once you are sick.* Don't wait until you are seriously
ill before changing your diet. As hard as it may seem to change your diet
now, it is much harder when you feel terrible. People with chronic disease
are often consumed with mere survival and following the doctor's orders,
which likely will not include healthy nutrition. People I know who are
seriously ill have no time, energy, or interest in any lifestyle change beyond
what their illness is forcing on them. It is often only after many years of
chronic disease that people are finally desperate enough to try a radical
change in diet. Why wait until you are desperate?

*Being healthy is appealing at every age.* Not every age group is motivated
by the potential to avoid disease, but there are good reasons why being
healthy can make a great difference in the quality of our lives, no matter
our age. Dr. John McDougall suggests that for children, a great motivator
is to avoid the pain and ridicule that can come from being, for example,
overweight or sluggish or having acne. For young adults, looking and feeling healthy is important to not only feeling good about oneself but also
attracting a mate. And of course, in the older years, delaying death and
disability are key motivators.

# Appendix 3

# Why Go 100%?

You may be thinking, do I really need to change my diet so radically? Wouldn't it be easier to improve my diet slowly, moderately, over time? If I stray from the diet here and there, will it really make that much of a difference?

The truth is there are many paths to a better diet. Kathy Freston, for example, recommends people "lean into" this diet. From her perspective, it doesn't matter so much how long it takes you to get to 100 percent, whether it is one day or one year (or even five years if you are young and healthy now). There are many paths. (If you are interested in this approach, check out her book *The Lean,* 2012.)

Most people prefer to make moderate changes over time, hoping the change will not be painful or take much effort. That is a fine way to go, if it works for you! I agree that each right choice and every effort we make to improve our diets is beneficial. Anything is better than nothing! But I'd like to present a few compelling reasons why you might consider going whole hog, cold-turkey, 100 percent on this diet within a relatively short time period (2–6 weeks).

No matter the path, it is important to have a compelling reason if you hope to radically change your diet. In this book, I've tried to present a compelling moral or religious reason, which is that the Word of Wisdom is a divine revelation from our Savior, who loves us and knows our bodies and spirits and thus knows what is best for us, and it is "pleasing" to Him when we eat this way. However, the fact is, most of the very righteous people around us do not eat this way, and, for many people, that one single fact can outweigh all the moral arguments. Science can certainly weigh in with strong evidence of the value of a whole food, plant-based diet, but if we want conclusive proof that doing this diet 100 percent is significantly healthier than 95 percent or 90 percent, we are not going to find it. Nutritional science is not that exact, and it is just as likely we'd find that 95 percent does not result in any health difference. But, there is another set of facts that make going 100 percent on this diet wise, even if the moral or scientific reasons are not compelling enough to us. That is what is explored here.

*Rich foods are addicting.* I'll start with interesting research which explains the impact of rich foods and why it is almost impossible for us to maintain a healthy weight when they are a part of our diet. Below I *summarize* some of the important points made by Doug Lisle and Alan Goldhamer in *The Pleasure Trap*, but the entire book is very worthwhile.

There are scientific explanations for why drug addicts have such a hard time quitting the habit. Our bodies are biologically designed to seek pleasure. Illicit drugs and substances like alcohol and tobacco artificially produce intense feelings of pleasure that are self-reinforcing. Not just people, but also animals, will abandon common sense and their own well-being to seek and obtain drugs. The feelings of pleasure are so intense and desirable that people will consume them for their short-term pleasure even though they often lead toward long-term unhappiness and ruin.

The highly processed, calorically dense foods produced by the food industry today are designed to trigger similar pleasure signals in our brains. The food industry knows how to produce products that are intensely pleasurable to us and will drive us to purchase them. As with drugs, we sometimes abandon common sense and even our own well-being by purchasing and consuming these foods. Eating rich, calorically dense food is a low-grade addiction for humans, similar in some respects to drugs. Like drugs, they provide short-term happiness that may rob us of our long-term joy and pleasure in life.

There are triggers in our bodies, as in all animals, that are biologically designed to help us eat the right amount of food each and every day. They are designed to tell us when we need more food and when we have had enough. When we are eating foods that our body is naturally designed to consume, these triggers work well. Even if animals have access to huge food resources, they do not consistently overeat. There are no obese animals living in the wild (just pets fed by humans!). So why are these triggers not working for us? Why do we overeat?

Even when we have eaten our fill, and we know we are full, we are driven to further consumption due to the pleasure signals the food triggers in us. Of course, we do not always get ever-increasing pleasure from food with further consumption. Our tastes adapt to the richness of the food, and the level of pleasure decreases, driving us to seek even more intensely rich foods to satisfy the low-grade addiction we've developed.

In addition, because the foods we are consuming are unnaturally rich and dense in calories, they fool the biological triggers in our bodies. All-important fiber, nutrients, and water have been taken out of the foods. Additional fat, sugar, and salt are added to them. This condition is so unnatural that our bodies have not adapted to it. Under these circumstances, our bodies are not able to accurately detect and tell us when we have had enough to eat. So, we continue to consume calories beyond the point that is good for us.

In short, as long as we are eating rich food that is unnatural to our bodies, we will be driven to eat more of it than is good for us and become overweight. If we eat less, we are inevitably left unsatisfied. So, we are trapped between feeling unsatisfied or being overweight. The only permanent way out is to eat the foods our bodies are designed to consume. If we do that, the biological triggers in our bodies work correctly to let us know when we need more food and when we are satisfied. We can then eat until we are satisfied and not gain weight. In fact, we will lose weight until we are at our ideal weight.

*Moderation is too hard.* What if instead of asking us to completely give up the most addictive substances, God simply counseled, "Tobacco, alcohol, and drugs are not good for you, so I advise you to use them moderately." How well would that work? Sometimes it is easier to "Just say no" than to try to figure out how much/little of it you'll eat each day. If we completely exclude foods that are not good for our bodies, we don't need to count calories, carbs, fat grams, or points, or worry about portion control.

Dr. John McDougall wrote:

> Westerners are completely addicted to their steaks, cheeses, and pies. Attempts at moderation guarantee continued dependence and continued failure. "Everything in moderation" has been preached to every generation throughout human history. Didn't work way back then and it doesn't work for folks today.
>
> Have you ever met a smoker who quit by cutting down?—I haven't. Have you ever heard of an alcoholic who sobered up by switching to beer?—neither have I. These moderate approaches keep the addicting agent within easy reach. The

only effective means to overcome these destructive habits is to remove the powerful substance from a person's life—repeated teasing with small fixes of the drugs (tobacco and alcohol) means unending torture and a quick return to the usual levels of use to avoid the pain.

Cutting down on the portion size of fried chicken, gravy, biscuits, and ice cream is slow torture and is one of the primary reasons diets fail. Simply put, these high-fat, high-salt, high-sugar foods are just too attractive for most mortals to resist.

This is the way Mary McDougall explains it:

Every positive experience you have with safer eating is important in getting you to the day when you do decide that you are worth the effort and finally going to make the change. You may decide to start slowly by slipping in an occasional [WFPB] recipe along with your old favorites. There's nothing wrong with this approach, except for a lot of heavy competition from those long-time favorite (and heavy) foods. Taking a part-way approach can set you up to suffer slow withdrawal symptoms—and inevitable disappointment in your results. You should not expect to gain the dramatic improvements in your health and appearance that the Program offers those who follow it strictly. When they're given no other choice, most people adjust to the new tastes and methods of food preparation within three or four days.

*Going 100 percent might actually be easier.* Dr. Colin Campbell answers the question, "Do you advocate a 100 percent plant-based diet?"

We eat that way, meaning my family, our five grown children and five grandchildren. We all eat this way now. I say the closer we get to a plant-based diet the healthier we are going to be.

It's not because we have data to show that 100 percent plant-based eating is better than 95 percent. But if someone has been diagnosed with cancer or heart disease, it's smart to go ahead and do the whole thing. If I start saying you can have a little of this, a little of that, it allows them to deviate off course. Our taste preferences change. We tend to choose the foods we become accustomed to, and in part because we become addicted to them, dietary fat in particular.

If we go to a plant-based diet, at first it might be difficult, but it turns out after a month or two our taste preferences change and we discover new tastes and feel a lot better, and we don't want to go back. It's not a religion with me, it's just that the closer we get to a 100 percent plant-based diet, the better off we're going to be.

Janice Stanger writes in *The Perfect Formula Diet*:

*Major shifts in eating patterns are easier for many people to follow than are small changes.* When you totally revamp your foods, your taste buds change their preferences within a few weeks. If you continue to eat your old favorites, even in small amounts, your old tastes are still being nurtured.

And I found this statement by an average person eating a WFPB diet:

I believe it's easier to follow the plan 100 percent than 95 percent. The cravings and obsessive food thoughts go away after a couple of months. You no longer have to struggle with [deciding to eat] a little bit of this or that off plan or feel bad when you indulge in SAD [Standard American Diet] food. People stop asking you if you want SAD food because they know you always say no.

*Dramatic changes lead to dramatic results.* If you want small changes in your health, make small changes to your diet. If you want big changes to your health, make big changes to your diet. If you want to reduce your chance of chronic illness, make small changes in your health. If you want to eliminate the chance of getting many of the common chronic illnesses, completely change your diet. This is from the blogger, The Healthy Librarian, who offers the following as "The Best Advice I Ever Got—Too Bad It Took Me Nine Years to Follow It":

You can ease into this—or jump into it 100 percent. But, let me warn you. If you ease into it—it will take you a long time to see the benefits. And you'll probably lose interest and quit before you get to that point. If you do it 100 percent you'll quickly see changes in your body & how you feel—and that will motivate you to keep it up. And you'll be able to more quickly lose the cravings for fatty, salty, & sugary foods.

According to the Monell Chemical Senses Study you will actually down regulate your fat receptors when you eliminate fat from your diet. You will stop craving it & wanting foods made with fat. The "fat craving" takes 90 days to go away. . . . The Esselstyn Diet works because if you follow the simple rules, you can't make a bad decision. Esselstyn has already removed the "bad guys" from the decision-making process. You don't have to waste time deciding *what not to eat*. Plus, you stay full—your blood sugar stays steady—and if you're smart, you've eliminated all the "bad guys" from your pantry & fridge.

There are at least two strategies for going 100 percent. The first is to begin, relatively soon, to go 100 percent for at least a definite period of time. Even if you don't stick with the diet, perhaps the most important reason to start now and go 100 percent is so you will learn what you (or someone you love) needs to do if you are ever in a position where you feel highly motivated to dramatically improve your health. At least try the diet for a long enough period so you learn how to feed yourself and enjoy the food. This could take as little as 21 days or as long as three months. You may later choose to discontinue the diet, but by then you will have learned enough to know how to make the change should you ever feel it is critical to do so.

The second strategy is to make it a goal to reach and stay at 100 percent. In this case, whether you reach that goal quickly or relatively slowly is less important than the fact that you are aiming at 100 percent and have a definite time frame to get there.

For more help on getting started, see: discoveringthewordofwisdom. com/getting-started/

# Appendix 4

# Guidelines for an Optimal WFPB Diet

The following guidelines are based on the work of Drs. Caldwell Esselstyn and John McDougall and registered dietician Jeff Novick. Even if you do not follow all these guidelines exactly, you will find it useful to know what they are so you can make better choices. See also: discoveringthewordofwisdom.com/wfpb-guidelines.

| Foods to Eat | Lots of nutrients! Enjoy a nice variety. |
| --- | --- |
| Grains and other starch foods in whole food form | Starches (complex unrefined carbohydrates) are the foundation of a good diet. They should be the bulk of your calories. Remember, "All grain is ordained… to be the staff of life." Eat WHOLE grains, the more unprocessed the better. For processed foods, the first ingredient on the label should be the word *whole* (100% stone-ground wheat is not whole wheat unless the word *whole* appears). Other whole grains include brown or wild rice, oats, wheat berries, rolled wheat, quinoa, etc. (If weight is an issue, limit flours, even those made from whole grains.) Other starches include roots (potatoes, yams, parsnips, etc.), winter squashes, beans, lentils, and peas. See http://www.drmcdougall.com/free_4b.html |
| Vegetables | For maximum weight loss, make vegetables one-third to one-half of your meal. Eat high-fat vegetables sparingly: avocados (88% fat); coconut (92% fat); and olives (98% fat). |

| Whole fruits | Whole fruits are far superior to processed fruits (e.g. applesauce, juices, smoothies, and/or dried fruits), but you might limit even whole fruits for weight loss or high triglycerides. |
| Legumes (beans, peas, and lentils) | Soybeans are higher in fat; eat more sparingly. |
| Herbs & Spices | These add variety and flavor. |
| **Foods to Avoid** | **The bad far outweighs any good.** |
| No meat, no poultry, no fish | Meat contains lots of saturated fat and cholesterol. It has too much protein (which can damage the liver and kidneys and increase the rate of cancer growth). Meat has few nutrients, no carbs, and no fiber. There is nothing in meat you can't get from a better source. |
| No dairy of any kind, not even skim milk or non-fat yogurt | The human body has no need for dairy (not even ice cream!). Dairy has the same problems as meat. While the non-fat versions don't contain the harmful fats, they contain an even higher concentration of animal proteins. Whole plant foods contain more than enough calcium for the human body. |
| No eggs, not even egg whites or Egg Beaters | Eggs have the same problem as meat and dairy. Your body does not need everything needed to grow a baby chick. |
| No oil (not even extra virgin olive, coconut, or canola oil) | The human body *does* need fat, but every plant naturally contains fat (where does the vegetable oil come from, after all?). Since plants contain the right amount of fats for our bodies, adding extra fat in the form of free oils just goes straight to our hips and bellies. Cooking spray labeled as zero calories and fat-free is 100% fat! (The FDA allows companies to round down to zero.) Non-stick cookware, parchment paper and silicone mats can be used effectively in place of cooking spray. Saùté with water instead. |
| Limit highly refined, processed foods | In general, the more a food is processed, the less nutritious it is. Be careful what processed foods you buy and use them sparingly. See the guide to reading labels later in this appendix. |

| Use Judiciously | Some of these are nutritious but contain negative elements. |
|---|---|
| Limit sugars | Limit the amount of sugar you consume to 5% or less of total calories. Maple syrup, agave, and honey are still sugar. Fruit juice and dried fruits are also very high in sugar. |
| Limit fruit juice | Eat your foods; don't drink them. Fruit juice is not the same as whole fruit, even if it is fresh or 100%. A little juice used to sauté or season recipes or for salad dressings is fine. Smoothies are a tasty treat, but it is even better to eat the whole fruits and veggies. Pure veggie juice is better because vegetables are low in sugar. |
| Limit soy products | Vegan soy products you find at the store are high in fat (40% +) and many are highly processed. "Fake foods" made from soy (soy burgers, soy turkey, etc.) are made from soy isolates, which are not healthy and should be avoided. Stick with traditional soy foods (tofu, soy milk, tempeh, miso, edamame, etc.) and avoid the fake soy products altogether. |
| Limit nuts, nut butters, seeds, and seed butters | There is a reason nuts have hard shells. Yes, they have nutrients and fiber, but they also have lots of fat (75–92%) and therefore calories. People with heart disease should eliminate nuts completely. Others should limit to no more than about an ounce per day. (Walnuts may be a better choice because of their omega 3 to omega 6 ratio.) |
| Limit high-fat plant foods | High-fat plant foods include avocados (88% fat); coconut (92% fat); and olives (98% fat). Don't over-eat these. If you have heart disease, eliminate them. Like nuts, they have lots of nutrients but also lots of fat. Other plants have the same nutrients without all the fat. If weight is an issue, just eliminate them. |
| Limit salt | You can safely eliminate salt from recipes (unless you are baking) and add it only at the table. Salting the surface of your food, which comes in direct contact with your taste buds, will enhance the taste while contributing far less sodium to your diet. |

| Limit for maximum weigh loss | Consuming too much can impede weight loss. |
|---|---|
| Flour products | Dry flour products, even those made from whole grains (whole grain bread, tortillas, pita, bagels, etc.) are more calorically dense than whole grains cooked in water or pasta. (To *gain* weight, eat *more* of these products.) |
| Dried fruits | Again, these are far more calorically dense than whole fruits and contain a lot of sugar. Whole fruits are better for you. |
| Fruit | Fruits are very nutritional, but they also contain a lot of sugar, so if you are trying to lose weight, better not to go hog wild on these. Some experts say for maximum weight loss, limit to 2–3 servings a day. Excess fruit sugars can raise triglycerides in some people. |

## Supplements to Consider

If you consume no animal products or foods fortified with Vitamin B12, plan to occasionally take a **Vitamin B12** supplement (you cannot overdose on this vitamin). 500 mcg/day is more than enough.

If you don't get enough sunshine (most of us don't) you might consider taking a **Vitamin D** supplement.

Some people take 1–2 tablespoons of *ground* **flaxseed** a day (store in the refrigerator) to increase omega-3 fats. This is optional.

A WFPB diet will provide all other vitamins and minerals. If you take additional supplements, you may not just be wasting money, you may be getting too much of a certain nutrient, which is not always a healthy thing to do. Nutrients are packaged ideally only in whole plant foods.

## What About Organic, Non-GMO, and Local?

A great many factors influence the amount of nutrients in a particular plant food, as well as how well your body absorbs the nutrients. The main point to remember is that whole plant foods are so full of nutrients that you don't need to worry about squeezing every last nutrient out of the plant and into your body! If some of the plant foods you eat are somewhat deficient in nutrients, it doesn't matter—unless your entire diet is poor.

The most important factor in your diet is whether you are consuming whole plant foods or crowding them out with animal/junk foods. In my experience, too many people pay far too much attention to whether their food is organic, fresh from the farm, not cooked or lightly cooked, compared with whether it is a whole plant food versus an animal food or processed food. The current epidemic of obesity and chronic disease is not caused by people consuming nonorganic vegetables! It is far better to eat overcooked, nonorganic, canned vegetables than to eat organic, grass-fed beef from so-called "happy" cows.

That said, organic foods have some advantages over nonorganic foods (though there are many other factors to consider: soil, freshness, seed quality, local conditions, cooking method, time in storage, etc.). Local produce is likely fresher than produce from South America. Lightly cooking food preserves some nutrients that will diminish if you boil the vegetables to death. But my advice is to not worry so much about these factors. Instead, concentrate on the most important factors: eating whole plant foods. If you have to worry you are losing nutrients because of the quality of the whole plant foods you buy or how you cook them, it probably means you are eating too many animal or processed foods and not enough whole plant foods. Once you have the basics down, if you have the time and money and interest to get extra fresh plant foods, go for it! If you don't, you'll be just fine.

## Plant Juices and Smoothies

I enjoy juices and smoothies as much as the next person, but I'm not crazy about them as staple sources of nutrition. Yes, these are easy ways to quickly consume a lot of plants, but are they the best way to consume food? Most of us don't need efficient ways to consume more calories. Humans did not evolve with fancy juicers and blenders. We are meant to chew our foods, with our mouths; it is supposed to take time. When high-powered machines process plants into tiny bits, it increases the surface area of these foods, which then interact with our bodies differently (increasing the insulin response, for example). Probably the worst thing about juices and smoothies is that people use them as "insurance," thinking they'll deliver all the nutrients they need so they don't need to worry so much about what they eat the rest of the day. Wrong. If you are eating right, you don't need the supposed extra nutrients from pulverizing plants. If you are not eating right, that is the place to focus your attention.

# Guide to Reading Food Labels—Based on the work of Jeff Novick, RD

Shop mainly in the produce section. When buying packaged foods, check for the following on the labels:

| Ingredient | Guideline |
|---|---|
| Fat | No more than 2.5 grams of fat per 100 calories (or no more than 20% of calories from fat). |
| | Avoid all saturated fats, hydrogenated fats, and tropical oils, including lard, butter, coconut, cocoa butter, palm oils, shortening, or margarine. Polyunsaturated fats (like safflower, soybean, corn, and sesame) and monounsaturated fats (such as olive and canola) are less harmful. If they are included, make sure the percentage of calories from fat is still 20% or less. |
| | Hidden fats: monoglycerides, diglycerides, triglycerides, lecithin, partially hydrogenated oils, myristic acid, suet. |
| Sugar | The less sugar, the better (none in the first three ingredients). Limit consumption of all concentrated caloric sweeteners to no more than 5% of calories in a day. At 5% of calories, which sugar you use will matter little to most anyone. |
| | Jeff Novick says, "Watch out for sugars and other caloric sweeteners that don't say 'sugar' but in fact are, such as corn syrup, rice and maple syrup, molasses, honey, malted barley, barley malt, or any term that ends in 'ol,' such as sorbitol or maltitol, or 'ose,' such as dextrose or fructose. Try to limit all these added, refined, concentrated sugars to no more than 5 percent of total calories (essentially, no more than 2 tablespoons daily for most folks). Don't be concerned about naturally occurring sugars . . . however, on the Nutrition Facts label, added sugars and naturally occurring sugars are all lumped together as 'sugar.' Your best bet: Look at the ingredient list. Try to avoid foods with added, refined caloric sweeteners in the first three to five ingredients. Because ingredients are listed in descending order of weight, the lower down the label you find added sugars, the better." |

| Salt | Try to not go over a 1:1 ratio of sodium mg to calories. That is, the amount of sodium in milligrams should be no more than the number of calories. If calories are 100, sodium should be no more than about 100 mg. Condiments can have more, if they are used sparingly. |
| --- | --- |
| Whole Foods | Buy less-processed foods, containing just a few ingredients which should be recognizable (not chemical-sounding names). One of Michael Pollan's "Food Rules" is, "Don't eat anything your great-grandmother wouldn't recognize as food." |
| Breads & Pastas | The first word should be "whole" (i.e., whole [name of grain] or stone-ground whole [name of grain]). These are also whole grains: brown rice, oats, oatmeal (including old-fashioned oatmeal), and wheat berries. Instant oatmeal is a whole grain but is more processed so is not as nutritious. The simplest bread contains flour, water, yeast, and salt, though other ingredients may be added. |
| Hidden animals foods | Ideally, eat whole non-processed foods, as they will not contain hidden animal byproducts. You may not choose to eliminate every bit of animal byproducts from your diet, but learn what they are, so you know what you are consuming.<br><br>Hidden dairy: caramel color or flavoring (*sometimes* derived from dairy), casein, caseinate, ghee, hydrolysates, lactalbumin, lactose, lactate, nougat, whey<br><br>Hidden egg: albumin, globulin, livetin, lysozyme, mayonnaise, meringue, ovalbumin (and anything beginning with ovo), silici albuminate, Simplesse, vitellin<br><br>Other animal foods: gelatin, rennet, carmine, isinglass, pepsin |

Ignore all the "health" claims stated anywhere on the packaging. They are almost always misleading.

Read the labels, especially THE INGREDIENTS!!!

## Additional Resources by Jeff Novick

Jeff Novick is a master teacher and has created many useful resources. Here are two on food labels you can find by searching the Internet:
"Understanding Food Labels"
"Identifying Hidden Sources of Salt/Sodium, Oil/Fat & Sugars/Sweeteners"

See also Jeff's excellent DVDs on shopping for food:
*Should I Eat That? How to Choose the Healthiest Foods*
*Fast Food - Vol 3: Shopping School*

Additional DVDs:
www.jeffnovick.com/RD/DVDs.html

## Updated WFPB Guidelines

These guidelines are kept updated at: discoveringthewordofwisdom.com/wfpb-guidelines.

# Appendix 5

# The Easy Way to Eat WFPB

If you already feel very comfortable in the kitchen, this appendix may not be as useful to you. The following strategies may be helpful to people like me, who start with limited cooking skills and who have limited time to figure out how to come up with delicious WFPB meals every day (see more ideas at: discoveringthewordofwisdom.com/wfpb-made-easy).

There are many strategies for preparing a healthy WFPB diet and thousands of recipes. Some recipes are easy, others much more complex, but what if you don't want to use any recipes? Here are simple suggestions.

**Breakfast** is easy: hot whole grain cereal with fruit and a non-dairy milk (with a little sweetener if needed). For savory breakfasts, add greens or cook up a quick dish of veggies.

**Lunch and dinner.** This is a simple formula:

1. Choose a starch.
2. Add whatever vegetables you like.
3. Use sauces and/or spices.
4. Have a piece of fruit for dessert.

## More Details on a Simple Lunch and Dinner Formula

**Choose a Starch.** The bulk of your calories should come from starches (whole complex carbohydrates). Be sure you have enough so you don't go hungry. You only need one starch for each meal (choose more only if you want). You can eat the same starch for each meal (or try a variety if you prefer). Here are some examples:

- *Whole Grains*: barley, oats, brown rice, quinoa, buckwheat, rye, bulgur (cracked wheat), triticale, couscous (refined wheat), wheat berries, corn, wild rice, millet

  Any of these work, but most work better as a breakfast cereal. I prefer rice or quinoa for lunch and dinner. A good rice cooker is worth every penny.

- *Roots*: burdock, sweet potatoes, celeriac (celery root), tapioca, Jerusalem artichoke, taro root, jicama, water chestnuts, parsnips, white potatoes, rutabaga, yam

  Potatoes and yams are familiar and easy to fix. Cook on the stove or in the oven. You can also wrap them in a slightly moist towel and microwave for about 5 minutes.

- *Winter Squashes:* butternut, acorn, hubbard, banana, pumpkin, buttercup, turban squash

  These can be steamed on the stove-top, cooked in the micro-wave, or baked in the oven.

- *Legumes*: **Beans** (aduki, red kidney, black, mung, fava/broad, navy, garbanzo, pink, great northern, pinto, limas, white kidney/cannellini); **Lentils** (brown, red, green); **Peas** (black-eyed, split yellow, split green, whole green)

  I enjoy adding beans to whatever other starch I have chosen. You can buy them in cans (choose low-sodium) or frozen or cook them yourself (cook in large quantities and freeze in small bags).

**Add Vegetables.** Add one or more vegetables to your liking. There are so many to choose from. Try to vary them week-by-week for different nutrients. Easy ways to cook them are as follows:

- Sauté without oil (use water, vegetable broth or any other non-oil liquid).
- Steam on the stove.
- Microwave (you can use any container, but I like using a silicone container with a lid).
- Roast in oven (instead of oil, try balsamic vinegar, oil-free sauce, or juice).
- Boil in water (you lose more nutrients this way, but you should be eating so many vegetables that the nutrients you lose won't make a difference health-wise).
- Eat them raw. You can add a good oil-free dip.

How to sauté onions without oil

- Use a good non-stick pan (like Berndes or Swiss Diamond) or a high quality regular pan (and watch it more carefully). Let it get hot.
- To hot, dry pan, add chopped onion and allow it to start to brown. It may appear to stick a little but let it get brown and caramelize without adding any water (otherwise you will start poaching the onion instead of sautéing).
- Once it starts to get brown, add a couple of tablespoons of non-oil liquid (e.g. water, juice, broth) but not too much (to avoid cooling the pan). The water added will bubble and steam.
- Immediately mix the onions around the pan with a non-metal spatula, using the small amount of water just added to collect the brown, caramelized contents from the sides of the pan.
- Add another couple of tablespoons of water to the pan and repeat the same process until the onions are brown and caramelized.

**Use Sauces and/or Spices.** Experiment with different spices and spice mixes (like Mrs. Dash or Table Tasty Salt Substitute). If you want to use salt, try to use little or none while you are cooking and then add a little to your food just before you eat.

You can make your own sauces (there are lots of recipes), but if you don't want to fiddle with recipes, there are many you can buy. Most sauces contain too much sugar, salt, or oil, so study the label carefully when you buy them. However, since they are used as a condiment (sparingly), don't worry if they contain a little more salt or sugar than you'd normally choose. Make sure there are no animal foods in the ingredients. Here are some sauces and flavorings you can easily find at the store:

- Salsa (there is such a huge variety out there, so experiment or make your own).
- Hot sauces (HUGE variety). Regular Tabasco sauce spices up any dish (try the various other flavors they have). Green taco sauce is also good.
- Mustard (again, many varieties).
- Vinegar (many, many varieties).
- Soy sauce, tamari, or Bragg's Amino Acids (get low-sodium varieties). For less sodium, try Raw Coconut Aminos (a soy

free, wheat free soy sauce with 113 mg of sodium per teaspoon) or low sodium miso (110 mg of sodium per teaspoon).

- Worcestershire Sauce (be sure it is vegan).
- A1 Steak Sauce
- Relishes

This **Walnut Sauce recipe** is as easy and delicious as they get. Almost everyone I know loves it. I use it on rice, potatoes, and any cooked vegetables.

---

### Walnut Sauce

Mix these ingredients in a food processor or blender:

- 1 cup walnut pieces
- 1 cup water
- 2–3 garlic cloves
- 2–4 tablespoons low sodium soy sauce or tamari sauce

---

**Enjoy Fruit for Dessert.** Once you have stopped eating sugary desserts, the fruit will taste sweet and satisfying.

## Other Quick Ideas

*If you are not trying to lose weight quickly*, you can also use whole grain, unrefined flour products: bread, pita bread, tortillas, pastas, etc. Use them to wrap some veggies, rice, beans, etc.

**Sandwiches.** Get good whole grain bread with little or no added oil. Add your favorite veggies. Mustard or non-fat hummus works great as a condiment.

**Tortillas.** Find whole wheat, brown rice, whole spelt, or corn tortillas. Add rice and beans to the veggies. Salsa works great, of course.

**Soup.** A good vegetable and/or bean soup can be very filling. This is great for weight-loss because of the amount of water.

**Pasta.** Use whole-grain as much as possible. Make sure there are no eggs in the pasta.

**Salad.** Choose your favorite veggies. Adding fruit works well. If you are used to traditional fat-filled dressings, it may take some time to get used to non-oil dressings. Don't worry: your tastes will change. Here is a simple no-oil salad dressing I make that has worked very well for me:

### 3-2-1 Salad Dressing

Mix these ingredients:

- 3 tablespoons balsamic vinegar
- 2 tablespoons mustard of choice (I use Dijon)
- 1 tablespoon maple syrup

## Snacks

Eating large meals will help cut down on the need to snack, but it is also good to have some healthy snacks around. Here are a few I like:

**Fruit.** This is the best! I especially love frozen grapes, YUM!

**Microwaved popcorn.** Put no more than ¼ cup of popcorn kernels into a small brown lunch bag; fold the top well, microwave until the popping slows way down. I like to spray some soy sauce on it for flavor. I sometimes also add some spices or nutritional yeast.

**Potato slices.** Microwave 5 minutes each side, or 20–25 minutes in the oven at 425°. Dip in no-oil hummus, salsa, or ketchup.

**Corn tortillas.** Cut into fourths, bake on a cookie sheet at 425° for ten minutes. Dip in salsa.

**Raw veggies.** Dip in a no-oil hummus.

**Cold cereal.** Choose a whole grain cereal with low sugar/fat.

## What I Eat

I am not a cook. I really mean that. You cannot be a worse cook than I. If I can do this, ANYONE over the age of 12 can do this. There are many wonderful foods you can eat on this diet. My way is extremely simple, and it works for me. Here is what I normally eat:

**Breakfast**: a whole grain, hot cereal (cracked or bulgar wheat; 5, 7, or 10-grain cereal; rolled, Scottish, or steel cut oats; brown rice; quinoa, etc.). My favorite is steel cut oats. I top it with chopped fresh fruit and frozen banana for sweetening and use non-dairy milk. I am currently also adding ground flax seed. This is all so delicious that before I go to bed each night, I'm already looking forward to breakfast!

You can cook whole grain cereals in the microwave, a slow cooker, pressure cooker, or rice cooker. On stovetop: Bring 2–3 parts water to boil, add 1 part grain, and turn down heat to low as you stir; then cover and cook for at least 10 minutes without opening the lid (make sure you turn down the heat low enough that it won't boil over). With a very large pan, you can make enough cereal to last you quite a few days, then just reheat in the microwave each day. I make one big batch (6 cups of dry oats) a week and then microwave a HUGE serving every morning in a silicone container.

**Lunch and Dinner**: My meals usually have three parts:

**A starch**. I make a starch item the center of each meal. My favorite is different varieties of brown rice. I cook a large batch in a top-of-the-line Asian rice cooker. The cooker does make a difference. Get an Asian brand, like the Korean Cuckoo.

**Beans**. I use a variety over time. Beans are inexpensive; buy low-sodium beans in cans (drain and rinse before using). They are even cheaper if you cook them yourself in a pressure cooker or slow cooker. I cook a big batch in a pressure cooker and then freeze them in small bags.

**Veggies**. These also vary widely, and I often have two to four kinds on my plate, though one is enough. I typically steam or sauté them, but they can also be boiled, roasted, or microwaved. You can experiment with adding spices, but I'm not very good at that. I do like to sauté some garlic and onion in a little water or vegetable broth; then after it is cooked, I add the vegetable and continue to cook until done, maybe adding some low-sodium tamari (a Japanese soy sauce) and chili garlic sauce. Adding tomatoes also works for me since I like juicy foods.

I use no sodium or very low sodium ingredients and add no salt while cooking, but then I add salt freely once the food is on my plate. I usually also use some "walnut sauce" on the veggies and/or beans and rice (see recipe above). I love to add fruit to my meals or eat afterward as dessert.

I also frequently have a very large salad for a meal (greens, a few veggies, garbanzo beans, fruit, etc.) with the 3-2-1 dressing (see above). I'm addicted to arugula!

I also eat other foods, but the above is my mainstay.

# Appendix 6

# Overcoming Challenges

While some people find it relatively easy to switch to a WFPB diet, most people should expect a challenge. Big change is usually difficult, and we should expect it to require dedication, persistence, a willingness to suffer some temporary discomfort, and a determination not to give up until we succeed.

Most things in life that are worthwhile take effort: getting an education, building a home, establishing a career, and raising children. Feeding ourselves appropriately is one of the important tasks of earth-life and is essential to our well-being, both physically and spiritually. Trying to figure this out is worthwhile, even if it takes some struggle and trial and error. Since Satan has a vested interest in our continuing to eat unhealthy foods that deaden our sensitivity to the spirit, expect and prepare for some opposition. But remember that the Lord cares even more what we eat, and He will certainly help us if we are determined and reach out to Him.

Once you are convinced that a WFPB diet is worth a try, you will face a number of challenges. These are probably the three biggest:

- Giving up certain foods.
- Figuring out what to eat.
- Dealing with other people.

Not every person faces all three challenges, but most do. Each challenge is difficult, and each takes time and effort to work through, but all can be overcome if you are willing to do what it takes to make it work. I provide here a few suggestions for meeting each challenge. This is a BIG topic, so I provide a lot more tips and advice from a variety of people on the website, discoveringthewordofwisdom.com.

# Giving Up Certain Foods

Humans can literally be addicted to the regular foods that are a normal part of the Standard American Diet: cheese, sugar, meat, fat, donuts. Overcoming these addictions can be very difficult. Here are three common approaches:

## Option 1: Go Cold Turkey

- Each time you taste food engineered to be highly pleasurable with excess fat-sugar-salt, you are dosing the dopamine-based pleasure receptors in your brain, which makes them crave more fat-sugar-salt laden food. Avoiding that altogether can be easier for many than having "just a little bit."

- Your sensitivity to certain tastes can change radically in just a few weeks. It takes 90 days for your "fat receptors" to down regulate.

- Clean out the refrigerator and pantry. If it's not possible to get rid of certain foods because other family members eat them, at least confine them all to one place/cupboard/shelf, etc.

- Commit to going cold turkey for a shorter timeframe than "forever." Twenty-one days is probably the shortest time that will still make a significant difference. Three months should kill off the worst cravings. Tell yourself, "It is just for three months, and then I'll re-evaluate."

## Option 2: Take Baby Steps

- A man who lost 300 lbs on a WFPB diet suggests that transitioning slowly can be easier for many than going cold turkey. He suggests that you make a list of everything you currently eat and then divide it into three categories: things you are going to completely eliminate this week/month (pick a time period); things you are going to reduce during this time period; and things you are not going to worry about during this time period. When you've got that list mastered or that time period ends, re-do the list.

- Another strategy: Choose one food at a time to stop eating; then move on to your next goal. An example from one family: We first eliminated meat, but not chicken broth. Then we eliminated fresh milk, then yogurt, then cheese, then ice cream. THEN we eliminated chicken broth. Then we began decreasing the amount of salt we used, and stopped using sugar and oil. We're now transitioning away from other sweeteners.

## *Option 3: Find a Buddy*

- We are inherently social creatures and having the help and support of others can be critical. If possible, find a friend who is willing to try the WFPB diet with you. Keep in touch on a regular basis. Work together on your goals. Encourage each other to stay strong. Eat together and also find enjoyable non-food activities to do together.

- If you can't find someone who is willing to change his or her diet with you, find someone who is willing to be your "buddy" in supporting you. Commit to reporting to that person each and every day (in person, over the phone, email, or text). Just knowing you will have to report every day will help you to stay on track. If that person can encourage you and provide nonfood rewards, all the better!

- If you can't find someone locally, you can locate people online to help support you. Use the McDougall Discussion Board at http://www.drmcdougall.com/forums. Write a post describing your situation and asking for advice and help. You'll find others who can answer your questions, provide support, and inspire you with their own stories. You may want to report your progress every day or every few days until this new diet becomes your lifestyle.

- Another program you can do in conjunction with others is the 21-Day Kickstart program at http://www.21daykickstart.org.

- Check out the Food Addicts Anonymous website (http://www. foodaddictsanonymous.org). Their philosophy is, "Food Addiction is a biochemical disorder that occurs at a cellular level and therefore cannot be cured by willpower or by therapy alone. We feel that food addiction is not a moral or character issue. This Twelve Step program believes that food addiction can be managed by abstaining from (eliminating) addictive foods, following a program of sound nutrition (a food plan), and working through the Twelve Steps of the program. After we have gone through a process of withdrawal from addictive foods many of us have experienced miraculous life-style changes."

## Behavioral Strategies

Doug Lisle, PhD suggests the following strategies:

- Clean your room; keep your environment clean. Lay out your exercise clothes to remind you to exercise—exercise helps you stay on track with healthy eating.
- Eat something healthy FIRST. Research shows that taste doesn't influence willpower as much as blood glucose does. Doug says, "The power in willpower is glucose." Whenever you are tempted, instead of telling yourself you can't have the off-plan item, simply choose to eat something healthy *first*, then re-evaluate whether you still want that other thing.
- Go to bed on time—get enough sleep but not too much. Sleep has an impact on appetite and willpower.

More behavioral strategies:

- Use a chart to hold yourself accountable. It can be very satisfying to put a checkmark on your chart to indicate you didn't eat any chips (sugar, cheese, or whatever) that day.
- The second law of thermodynamics says that we tend to go from a state of order to disorder. This is true both spiritually and physically. We go to church and read scriptures as a way to keep our spirit from "disorder." We need to CONSTANTLY remind ourselves of why we make the health choices we make. You can do this by using books, websites, friends, and any other resource that keeps you motivated.

## Spiritual Strategies

- Elder Boyd K. Packer wrote, "True doctrine, understood, changes attitudes and behavior. The study of the doctrines of the gospel will improve behavior quicker than a study of behavior will improve behavior." Study the Word of Wisdom and other scriptures and good books.

- Identify why you are eating something unhealthy for your body. Are you too Hungry, Angry, Lonely or Tired (HALT)? Are you fulfilling an emotional need? Can you turn that over to the Lord and ask Him to fill you? Can you recognize the source of your craving and reaffirm that there is only one Source that will ever completely fulfill that need? (Hint: it's not food.)

- Ask yourself what it means to you that the Word of Wisdom was given for the "weakest of all Saints" (D&C 89:3)?

- Review 1 Nephi 3:7. Search other scriptures (you'll be amazed at what's in there that relates to this).

- Fast. Whether it is a 24-hour fast or simply fasting between meals, remember that one of the purposes of fasting is to bring your spirit back into control over your body. Take advantage of that. Study Elder Russell M. Nelson's excellent October 2013 General Conference address, "Decisions for Eternity." He says, "A pivotal spiritual attribute is that of self-mastery—the strength to place reason over appetite. Self-mastery builds a strong conscience. And your conscience determines your moral responses in difficult, tempting, and trying situations. Fasting helps your spirit to develop dominance over your physical appetites. Fasting also increases your access to heaven's help, as it intensifies your prayers."

## Resources on Overcoming Food Addictions

*The Pleasure Trap: Mastering the Hidden Force that Undermines Health & Happiness* by Douglas J. Lisle and Alan Goldhamer (2006)

*Breaking the Food Seduction: The Hidden Reasons Behind Food Cravings— And 7 Steps to End Them Naturally Paperback* by Neal D. Barnard (2003)

Video: http://nutritionfacts.org/video/changing-our-taste-buds/

## Understanding the Food Industry's Role in Addiction

*Salt Sugar Fat: How the Food Giants Hooked Us* by Michael Moss (2013)

*The End of Overeating: Taking Control of the Insatiable American Appetite* by David A. Kessler (2010)

*Your Food Is Fooling You: How Your Brain Is Hijacked by Sugar, Fat, and Salt* by David A. Kessler (2012)

*Mindless Eating: Why We Eat More Than We Think* by Brian Wansink (2010)

# Figuring Out What to Eat

Figuring out how to eat a good plant-based diet is difficult for several reasons: (1) our taste buds are accustomed to meat and processed foods, so it takes time to learn to appreciate whole foods; (2) cooking whole foods inevitably takes longer, especially at first, so we have to readjust our thinking and habits; (3) learning a new way of cooking takes time; (4) everyone's tastes and habits are different so there is not "one system" that works for everyone—others can provide ideas, but you have to work out the solutions on your own.

With this diet, you will primarily be cooking from scratch—there is really no way around it. Unless you can afford to hire a cook or know someone who will cook for you, you will be doing a lot of cooking. There will be few, if any, local restaurants you can rely on.

Even though it takes effort, you can do it, especially if you decide you're going to keep working until you succeed. I know it is do-able because I started with literally zero cooking skills, and I was able to figure it out. I can now feed myself relatively quickly, and I *very* much enjoy my food. (I admit, however, it is harder if you have to feed someone else who is eating differently!)

You can find literally thousands of free recipes online. Of course, you don't need thousands; you don't need more than 7–12 basic foods to create a weekly menu, but you may need to explore several dozen items before you figure out what you like and what works for your lifestyle.

## One Strategy for Finding Foods You Will Like

- Make a list of all the foods you currently enjoy that already fit within the guidelines of this diet.
- Add to that list any foods you like that you can make fit the guidelines with minimal adjustments.
- Try recipes in books and/or online to find additional foods you enjoy—ones that work for you in terms of taste and preparation time.

- After you have a basic set of 6–7 recipes you like, continue to make them each week. You may want to make a detailed weekly menu so you can get all your shopping done at one time and be prepared for the full week. Make large batches so you don't need to cook every day.
- As you have time and interest, try a new recipe.

Keep it simple. You can find foods you like before you begin the diet, or stick to a few foods that you already know how to make while you explore new recipes.

## Practical Suggestions

- Clear out your fridge and cupboards of all non-compliant foods, or if that is not possible, stick them in a place where you can't see them unless you make a concerted effort.
- Stock up on staples that can last awhile: cans of low-sodium beans; whole grains and other starches; frozen fruits and veggies; spices and condiments.
- Make a menu plan. Do produce preparation on shopping day so that you have already chopped/prepped veggies for a quick meal.
- Be sure to eat enough food every day so you are not hungry. If you are hungry you will be tempted to eat something unhealthy. If you eat until you are full at each meal, you'll do much better. Be prepared: on this diet, the volume of food will be larger than what you ate before. However the cost, especially if you buy in bulk and prepare most foods at home, can be much cheaper—in some areas of the country as low as three or four dollars per day.
- Have some healthy snack foods available when you need something extra or want to munch on something. Keep some healthy snacks in your car, office, or anywhere else you spend lots of time.
- Cook food in large quantities and eat leftovers (or freeze for later).
- Experiment with spices to flavor your food. It may take a while to figure out what you like.
- Join a Kickstart program where you'll be introduced to many types of food: http://www.21daykickstart.org.
- Remember, if you are not enjoying your food as much as before, don't panic. *This will not last forever, just a relatively short time period.* Not enjoying your food for a few weeks is NOT the end

of the world. We humans are designed to enjoy wholesome plant foods; you will learn to love them!

## Notes about Making the Transition

**It may take time for your body to adjust to more fiber.** If your diet does not currently contain a lot of *whole* grains, starchy vegetables, and legumes, your body has long since adjusted to a low fiber diet. Suddenly switching to a high fiber diet can cause abdominal bloating, stomach pain and/or intestinal gas in some people. If you are worried, just increase the fiber more slowly. Your body will definitely adjust over time and thank you for it!

**It may take time for your taste buds to realize how delicious this food is.** While many people love the foods on this diet from the start, we are so used to food with lots of fat, sugar, and salt that this diet can taste bland and uninteresting at first. It may take some time for your taste buds to change and for you to find what you like. You may need to experiment with seasonings. Be patient. Your taste buds WILL change, and you WILL figure out what to eat. You'll soon be enjoying every meal! Expect anywhere from 2–12 weeks.

# Dealing with Other People

In my experience, the social aspect of a WFPB lifestyle is the most challenging. Taste buds change, cooking skills improve, but it may take more time to learn how to deal with the great variety of social challenges that can make our chosen diet difficult to maintain. Fortunately, for a variety of reasons, people in our society are on all kinds of special diets, so we are not alone. In fact, you will find that many people will be sympathetic and will help you, even if they themselves are not on a special diet. There are certainly many ways to present your "new self" to the world. Here are just a few:

**Be loud.** Announce to everyone what you are doing and ask for support. If you have any health concerns, you can use them as an excuse and a reason to ask others to help you make this transition. Make it clear that you are now eating a different way, and tell all of your family and friends so they will know in advance to not be surprised when you don't want a slice of the apple pie they just baked (in fact, they'll know not to offer it to you).

**Be quiet.** Don't say anything and try to blend into the crowd. Eat before you go out, and when you are eating with a group, eat only what is acceptable to you, but eat very slowly and engage actively in the conversation (even if you are just listening well to what others are saying). You'll be surprised how few people notice you aren't eating much. If someone says something, have a ready comment to make that is both simple and honest:

- "I've had plenty. Thanks so much!"
- "I'm not very hungry today."
- "I've overeaten all this week, so I'm cutting back."
- "I am trying to lose weight."
- "I have a health condition, so I'm trying to be careful."

If someone makes an issue of your diet, and it isn't the right time or place to discuss it (or you don't want to), you can downplay it and make it a non-issue: "Yes, it is a pretty crazy diet. Who knows how long it will last!"

**Be a missionary**. This is my favorite strategy. If anyone notices what I'm eating, I use it as an opportunity to express my joy in my new diet. If they have a moment and look interested, I tell them my story. If they ask questions, I answer them. If they express an interest, I send them more information later.

**Be passionate**. This is similar to being a missionary, but rather than trying to convert others, you are simply sharing your joy of eating this way. If anyone asks, let them know you love the food, love the way you feel, and love the things you are learning. You don't want to make others feel guilty about the way they eat (we were all there!), just express that you are having a great adventure.

**Be a pioneer**. If you joined the LDS Church as an adult, you already know all about this. Family and friends are not always happy when we make big changes in our lives that don't include them. But if we are kind and patient, stick to our commitments, and continue to love them, they will soon respect our decision. They may begin to defend us in front of others, and someday they may even join us! If it is not easy to be a pioneer, take comfort in the fact that what you are doing is important work that is actually needed by those who are currently not supporting you. Some day they may thank you.

**Be an individual**. In this approach, you are careful to let others know that you know there are many paths to eating healthily, but you feel good about the path you are on; you feel this is the right path for you at this time in your life. If someone challenges you, you can just say, "It seems to be working for me right now." Recognize that others feel good about moving in different directions, and that is fine with you.

**Be yourself.** Relax. You don't need to impress or persuade anyone. Be real, sincere, and genuine, and you'll find people readily accepting the changes you have made.

## Specific Situations

**Young children.** Children under a certain age don't have much choice (and probably should not be given a lot of choice) in what they eat at home. Children can adapt surprisingly well. You have less control when your children are outside of your home. However, being too strict often backfires. Teach correct principles, and they can learn by making some of their own decisions.

**Older children.** Teens and young adults need to be able to choose. Compelling older children to eat a certain way may not be wise. On the other hand, life will be simpler at home if you are cooking just one meal. If they want to eat differently, allow them to add meat, cheese, or butter to the meals you prepare or do some of their own cooking.

**Spouses and other adults.** Don't nag or complain. Each person must come to these decisions on their own. If you have traditionally cooked for your spouse, and your spouse doesn't want to change the way he/she eats, you will likely feel it is worth it to make variations of a recipe, one for the spouse and one for you. You can easily add meat or cheese to half of the recipe near the end of the cooking time (e.g. add meat to the salad or spaghetti sauce; add cheese to pasta). Your kindness and patience will pay off eventually!

**Eating at someone else's home.** Eat before you go so you are not hungry. Offer to take something to contribute to the meal. If necessary, let the host know you don't eat animal foods and suggest something simple you can eat: baked potato, rice, or salad (take your own salad dressing).

**Having guests at your home.** Once you learn how to cook WFPB food well, you'll be able to find foods that are also appealing to people eating a Standard American Diet. You may choose to add a few options you wouldn't normally have, like butter and a higher fat salad dressing.

**Church activities.** Again, eat before you go. If you can, find out what is being served and bring something comparable for your family to eat. If you quietly put it on the food table, labeled "vegan," the only people who notice are those who appreciate having it there.

If you are responsible for the food for a ward activity, GREAT! You can often separate the junk food from the nutritious food so that ward members can choose how much of the junk they want to consume.

Better yet, introduce the diet to others in the ward. If you are as fortunate as I have been, there will be enough people who want to eat WFPB that there will be plenty of WFPB options at the next ward or Relief Society pot luck. We even had a "vegan cookie table" at our Relief Society cookie night last year!

I personally have not had the experience of someone accusing me of NOT keeping the Word of Wisdom by not eating meat, but I understand others have. You might study the related scriptures in case they honestly desire to explore the issue with you, but otherwise, I suggest using humor and self-effacement. I sometimes refer to my diet as something "crazy" and "way out there" in order to not make an issue of it in social situations.

**Eating Out—Restaurants.** Research the menu online before you go, and find something you can eat. There usually are at least one or two things you can eat, though sometimes you may want to ask the chef to adjust the recipe (e.g. "Please don't add any oil when you cook this"). Most restaurants are very good at making accommodations. If you find nothing on the menu, you may be able to find basic ingredients you like in other menu items and then ask the chef to put them together. Asking doesn't hurt, especially if you do it in a very nice way. For a nicer restaurant, you may want to call a few hours ahead of time to give them a heads up.

## Remember, Remember

If making the switch is not easy, it is definitely worth it. Look at all the sick people around us. What is our health worth? Yes, eating this way is not always easy, but living with cancer or heart disease is not easy either. Believe me, if you get heart disease, you'll learn to live with it because you'll have no choice. I would rather freely choose to eat in a way to prevent heart disease in the first place.

I believe the problem is not knowledge; it is commitment. All the scriptures implore us to "remember." It is right there in the Word of Wisdom, "remember to keep and do these sayings" (D&C 89:18). We know what to do to take better care of our bodies, but it is easy for us to not "remember" to make the best choices. Perhaps one reason is that we feel we are only hurting ourselves. We don't remember that we are not our own, that we were "bought with a price" (1 Corinthians 6:19–20). And what a price that was. "Therefore," Paul admonishes, "glorify God in your body, and in your spirit, which are God's" (1 Corinthians 6:20). If we believe this, what will it take to help us remember?

Ultimately, health reasons may not be enough to help us remember. I do believe our ability to commit ourselves to eating well is greatly strengthened when we see it in light of our religion and commitment to God, when we do it because we have a testimony that it is pleasing to Him. Gandhi, a life-long vegetarian, wrote:

> Forty years ago I used to mix freely with vegetarians. . . . I notice also that it is those persons who became vegetarians because they are suffering from some disease or other—that is from purely the health point of view—it is those persons who largely fall back. I discovered that for remaining staunch to vegetarianism a man requires a moral basis.

Fortunately, we have the ultimate "moral" reason for eating a wholesome diet: an amazing revelation from God called the Word of Wisdom.

# Appendix 7

# Recommended Books, Resources, Recipes

Resources supporting a whole food, plant-based diet are abundant, and new resources are popping up all the time. More than you'll ever have time to fully explore is freely available on the Internet, but I recommend you include the following two items in your study, even if you have to purchase them.

1. *Forks Over Knives* (2011). This documentary is the best short introduction to a WFPB diet. It is widely available through Netflix, Hulu, Amazon, and possibly your local public library. Don't miss it.

2. *The China Study* by T. Colin Campbell and Thomas Campbell (2006). I think this is the best book on the subject. Campbell does not include practical advice or recipes, but he presents the main scientific facts in a compelling way, backing every assertion with appropriate references. It may be available at your local library, but I encourage you to purchase the book. It is inexpensive and well worth the cost.

## WFPB Websites and Related Resources

Due to the generosity of many WFPB experts, there is plenty of information freely available on the Internet. Below, I highlight a few favorite websites, especially from the long-time heavyweights in this field, but you can find plenty more if you look. I also describe a few more books and other resources featured on these sites.

### *Dr. John A. McDougall, MD* — drmcdougall.com

Dr. McDougall has been promoting a WFPB diet (which he calls a "starch-based" diet) longer than anyone on this list. His website is a treasure trove. It contains a huge variety of useful information, helpfully organized by topic. He provides a free program, free videos, excellent newsletters, hundreds of recipes, and a huge, very active, discussion board. He also sells very useful books, DVDs, seminars, and short-term live-in programs, but the basic information is entirely free (and completely adequate for achieving success). You can also find many more videos by Dr. McDougall on YouTube.

I also recommend Dr. McDougall's latest book, co-written with his wife, Mary McDougall, *The Starch Solution* (2012). It is the culmination of over 40 years of experience and contains much of the knowledge he and Mary have gained over the years through research, interactions with thousands of patients, and spreading the word about a low fat, starch-based diet through books, seminars, and other presentations. But frankly, all of McDougall's books contain the exact same message. He has not needed to change his advice because it is really that simple.

## Dr. Caldwell B. Esselstyn, Jr., MD — www.dresselstyn.com

This site features Dr. Esselstyn's excellent book *Prevent and Reverse Heart Disease: The Revolutionary, Scientifically Proven, Nutrition-Based Cure*. The book is well worth reading; if you would prefer not to make a purchase, there is plenty of free information on his site (see dresselstyn.com/site/articles-studies). You can also find many more videos by Dr. Esselstyn on YouTube. He is a great presenter, so be sure to watch at least one!

Dr. Esselstyn has worked with hundreds of patients, and he has documented the power of a WFPB diet to stop and reverse the progression of heart disease. He presents the medical evidence for abstaining from free oils in a clear, understandable fashion that will convince even the most reluctant readers of the importance of taking care of their endothelial lining.

## Forks Over Knives — forksoverknives.com

This growing website, based on the documentary with the same name, is worth subscribing to so you get free emails when it is updated. It contains great personal stories, good advice, and wonderful recipes.

## T. Colin Campbell, PhD — nutritionstudies.org

Colin Campbell is the author of the must-read book *The China Study*. See also his excellent new book, *Whole: Rethinking the Science of Nutrition* (2013). For people who really want to dive into the science behind a

WFPB diet, consider enrolling in his Certificate in Plant-Based Nutrition course offered through the T. Colin Campbell Foundation and eCornell.

### *Jeff Novick, MS, RD* — jeffnovick.com

Jeff Novick is an extraordinary teacher. You can check out clips from some of his presentations online, but his DVDs are worth purchasing. His *Fast Food* DVDs take you through the process of making quick, delicious, and nutritious food in ten minutes or less with items you can store in your pantry and freezer. In his series on weight loss and nutrition, he draws on his expertise as a plant-based dietician to help you sort fact from fiction in a world full of contradictory dietary advice.

Jeff moderates many of the discussion boards on Dr. McDougall's site, drmcdougall.com/forums, which makes these even more valuable. Also check out his Facebook page for a steady stream of news and good advice.

### *Rip Esselstyn* — engine2diet.com

Rip is Caldwell Esselstyn's son. His book, *The Engine 2 Diet* (2009) is a great read and is especially good for the young adult population. The website keeps it simple with essential basic facts and recipes and links to additional resources. Whereas Dr. Esselstyn's diet is considered "plant perfect," geared especially toward those who are recovering from heart-related events, Rip's advice is "plant strong" and will appeal to those in relatively good health who are looking for more energy and better performance.

### *Neal D. Barnard, MD* — pcrm.org — nealbarnard.org

Dr. Barnard is the Founder and President of the Physicians Committee for Responsible Medicine (PCRM). He is a long-time advocate of a WFPB diet and also a strong proponent of protecting animals. His books are all very well-written and useful. The PCRM website includes well-organized research on various topics, breaking news, and recipes.

### VegSource.com

This site, ably run by Jeff and Sabrina Nelson, links to a lot of useful resources. This site does not shy away from controversy, and you can find all kinds of interesting things here.

## *Dr. Michael Greger, MD* — nutritionfacts.org

Dr. Greger does an amazing job of summarizing and sharing peer-reviewed research data in an entertaining, useful way. Unfortunately, because most academic research is so reductionist, it is hard to interpret, and even with these helpful videos you'll find plenty of contradictory advice. I recommend two videos in particular:

"Uprooting the Leading Causes of Death," http://nutritionfacts.org/video/uprooting-the-leading-causes-of-death

"More Than an Apple a Day: Combating Common Diseases," http://nutritionfacts.org/video/more-than-an-apple-a-day-preventing-our-most-common-diseases

## *Dr. Joel Fuhrman, M.D.* — drfuhrman.com — diseaseproof.com

Dr. Fuhrman provides some good, solid information. His forum is only available to paid subscribers, and he sells a lot of things from his website. I'd stick with the free stuff. His book, *Eat to Live*, is a best seller and has been highly influential in converting people to a WFPB diet.

## Updated List of Resources

For an updated list of the best WFPB resources, including links to the Discovering the Word of Wisdom support groups and Facebook page, see: discoveringthewordofwisdom.com/more-resources

## Facebook.com

Of course, most of the experts have their own Facebook pages. If you love Facebook, you'll want to check out all of them. Here are a few:

www.facebook.com/DrJohnMcDougall
www.facebook.com/Dr.Esselstyn
www.facebook.com/JeffNovickRD
www.facebook.com/forksoverknives
www.facebook.com/drfuhrman

## Low-Fat Whole Food, Plant-based Recipes

There are literally *thousands* of low-fat WFPB recipes online. You only need a half dozen to a dozen that you really like. Don't get overwhelmed. Try a few here and there until you discover what you like! For an updated list, see: discoveringthewordofwisdom.com/links-to-recipes

**The McDougall Free Program.** This free program includes recipes to get you started (see link to the "10-Day Meal Plan"). www.drmcdougall.com/health/education/free-mcdougall-program

**McDougall Newsletter Recipe Index.** This is a massive database of recipes, more than you could ever make in a lifetime. www.drmcdougall.com/health/education/recipes/mcdougall-newsletter-recipes/

**The Cancer Project Recipe Index.** Plenty of gems. www.nutritionmd.org/recipes/all.html

**Fat-Free Vegan.** Hundreds of well-organized recipes. fatfreevegan.com

**Forks Over Knives Recipes.** Sign up for the newsletter for more recipes. www.forksoverknives.com/category/recipes

**Engine 2 Diet Recipes.** Find more great recipes in Rip Esselstyn's books. engine2diet.com/recipes

**Naked Food Magazine.** This is a new WFPB magazine: nakedfoodmagazine.com/category/nakedkitchen

**Examples blogs.** There are many more!
Marla's Marvelous Meals: www.vegsource.com/marla
Straight UP Food: www.straightupfood.com
Happy Herbivore: happyherbivore.com
Healthy Girl's Kitchen: www.healthygirlskitchen.com
Greener Eating: www.greenereating.com
New Paradigm Health Cookery: www.newparadigmhealthcookery.com/recipes
Helen's Healthy Kitchen: www.helynskitchen.com

**A few WFPB cookbooks.** I compiled this short list. www.amazon.com/lm/R3Q3UZL7A4HHXM

# About the Author

Jane Birch was born in 1961 and is the oldest of nine children. As a child, she always had her nose stuck in a book, so she probably missed a lot of what was happening, but she loved school, and life only got better when she entered Brigham Young University as a freshman in 1979. Jane served in the Taiwan Taipei Mission (1983–84) and has a great love for the Chinese people. She earned a BA in History (1986) and a PhD in Instructional Science (1994) at BYU.

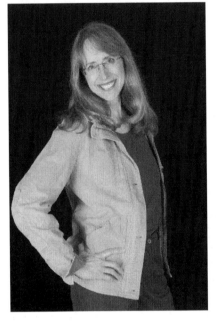

Jane is currently Assistant Director for Faculty Development at the BYU Faculty Center. She developed BYU's premiere faculty development program, an 18-month program for all new faculty. Her favorite part of her job is helping faculty explore the relationship between the gospel of Jesus Christ and their work as teachers and scholars.

Jane is wildly enthusiastic about books and all variety of learning. In addition to her passion for the Word of Wisdom and the whole food, plant-based lifestyle, she loves literature, philosophy, religion, history, and music. She also thoroughly enjoys great conversation, travel, working on her Apple Mac computers, and "organizing stuff." Lately, she is very interested in near-death experiences (reading them, not having them).

Jane's testimony of the gospel is her pearl of great price. She loves the plan of salvation and the opportunity each of us has to participate in something as grand as building the Kingdom of God on earth. She sincerely believes that "waking up" to the Word of Wisdom is a critical part of preparing the Saints for the last days and the coming of our Savior.

# About the Cover

I call my introduction to a whole food, plant-based diet, "an answer to a question I did not ask." I was not searching for ways to improve my diet.

I had no reason for or interest in changing the way I ate. But after learning about the WFPB diet, I was quickly convinced that this is the way humans are supposed to be eating, that this is in line with the Word of Wisdom, and that consequently I needed to be eating this way. It was an answer to a question I did not ask.

I immediately gave up all animal foods and junk foods—foods I had thoroughly enjoyed my entire life, foods I had never once considered giving up before that day. I have never looked back. It has been a joyful adventure ever since.

I have often reflected on why I made this huge change so quickly and so relatively easily. Why me? Why at this time? And why have I felt so motivated to introduce this diet to others? Why did I go on to write an entire book on the Word of Wisdom?

The day after learning about this diet, I asked my mom if she had the book *The China Study*, one of the most influential WFPB books. She did, and the copy she gave me was one that my uncle, Cliff Lamb, had read. He had marked the text and written in the margins. I loved reading it. *The China Study* had the same impact on me that it has had on thousands of others. I also felt close to my Uncle Cliff as I read this book, and since then, I have thought of him often.

Clifford Lamb died in 2010, just a year prior to my learning about this diet. He was a beautiful person and a very talented artist. He was also well known in the family for being extremely careful about eating a very healthy diet. He loved the Word of Wisdom and studied it often. He also loved *The China Study*. He gave a copy of this book to all his sisters, including my mother.

Because Cliff ate such a healthy diet, I remember feeling sad that I never had the chance to discuss my new diet with him, to let him know that I had joined him in being a healthy eater. I knew that would please him.

About eight months after changing my diet, I felt impressed to do more writing on the relationship between the Word of Wisdom and a whole food, plant-based diet. As I shared my writing with others, they encouraged me, and this idea gradually grew into a book-length project. Prior to this, I had always thought that writing a book would be a very painful undertaking, but writing this book was a joyful experience. The words just flowed. I felt greatly blessed.

While working on this book, I also happened to start reading many near-death experiences. Through my readings, I became much more aware of how close people in the next world are to the people in this world. I learned that there are angels all around us, helping us, and that they are usually people we know. I started to wonder if Cliff's influence could be a factor in my learning about this diet, in my continued interest in it, and in my writing a book. I began to think I might be receiving help from him and others from the other side.

Then a story I heard convinced me that the feelings I had about Cliff and this diet were not a coincidence. Kim Rives reported that while having a near-death experience and being in the next world, she was allowed to visit her sister in this world. She could see her sister, who was writing her thesis on her computer, but she could also see that there was a beautiful male angel standing right beside her. Her sister couldn't see her or the angel, of course. Kim describes watching the angel:

> He was helping my sister with her thesis. She was writing things on the computer, and then when he didn't like what she had written, he had his pen, and he would cross it out in red and without flicking it, he could write in gold, and he would write what he wanted her to write. She'd stop for a minute, you know, backspace, delete, and then she would write almost word for word what he had just written. One of the most amazing things, and I saw her do it over and over.

When I heard this, I immediately thought, "If an angel would help someone write her master's thesis, would not an angel help me write a book on the Word of Wisdom?" This certainly would explain why I have felt so driven, so blessed, and so helped in putting this work together. Time after time when I needed something, the way was opened, and ideas flowed into my mind.

After hearing this story, I was convinced I am not the only person involved in writing this book. I now believe there are others, possibly many others (both in this world and in the next), with an interest in this work, whose righteous desires are being fulfilled, in part, by what I'm doing. The help I've received has been so steady and so marvelous, I've come to expect it. This feeling has only increased as people have sent me their stories to include in the book, and I've been learning how Mormons all over the world are "waking up" to the Word of Wisdom and embracing a whole food, plant-based lifestyle.

When it came time to design the cover of this book, a cover artist prepared a few designs for me to consider, but none of them worked for me. I felt stumped and shared this with my mother. My mom suggested,

"Why don't you use the artwork Cliff did of the watermelon?" At first, this didn't seem possible, as Cliff's watermelon is oriented horizontally, and I couldn't picture it as a book cover. Then, a couple days later, I realized I could turn the watermelon on its side. Suddenly, it looked like a book cover! I added some text for the title and author and had a feeling that this was an answer to prayer.

When I shared this idea with Cliff's wife, my Aunt Janet, she was absolutely thrilled. She said, "This is exactly what Cliff wanted to have happen, to write a book like this." She said her kids often talk about how their dad taught them how to eat. They say, "He taught us two things: how to read the scriptures and how to eat." I said, "That is amazing because that is just what this book is about: how to read the scriptures we have that teach us how to eat."

After this conversation with my aunt, I composed the first draft of the words of gratitude to Cliff, which now appear on the dedication page of this book. As I did, I felt a great sense of joy and peace. I feel confident that Uncle Cliff is pleased that his artwork is now an integral part of this book. He truly was my angel in writing it. I feel we have written the book he wanted to write.

---

I love Cliff's depiction of a watermelon. By focusing on just one of the glorious plant foods ordained by God for our use, I believe Cliff invites us to look deeply into the beauty and mystery of wholesome plants. I hope this cover will inspire readers to ponder on the power of the foods God has blessed us with and to consider why they are ordained for our "constitution, nature, and use" (D&C 89:10). I hope it will encourage us to use them with "prudence and thanksgiving" (D&C 89:11). I also hope this cover will convey the message of breaking open the Word of Wisdom to find the deeper meaning, the most delicious fruit.

# Acknowledgments

While completing this book, I was inspired by Diana Nyad's successful swim from Cuba to Florida. One of the messages she shared as soon as she got to shore was, "It looks like a solitary sport, but it takes a team." This is equally true of writing a book. Fortunately, I had a great "team." My thanks to *everyone* who helped and supported me in any way!

First, thanks to Abbie Gyungsook Kim, who inadvertently introduced me to this diet and then became the best WFPB cook I know! A special thanks goes to my mother, Judy Birch, and sister, Elizabeth Rose. They immediately supported me in making this change, and they (and the rest of my family) have made it easy for me to eat WFPB at every family gathering.

I've made a lot of new friends through this diet who have greatly blessed my life. Mark and Saundra Gotberg were the first "McDougallers" I had the privilege to meet and learn from. Debbie Christofferson and Ilene Christensen are forever WFPB friends. Rogan Taylor wrote the foreword and has been a great partner and friend and graciously took my photo for this book. And Jessica Duffett is my new WFPB buddy.

My gratitude to all the great WFPB doctors and other experts who so generously share their expertise and experience with all of us, especially Colin Campbell, Caldwell Esselstyn, John McDougall, and Jeff Novick. The message they are teaching is plain and precious!

Special thanks go to Professor Paul Peterson. I never got a chance to share my enthusiasm for the Word of Wisdom with him, but I felt his, and I felt his spirit as I wrote this book. I am hopeful he is pleased with my effort.

I feel very blessed to have received the stories I got for this book and to work with all the wonderful storywriters! They not only contributed their work, they also helped with ideas for the book and provided feedback as it neared completion.

A BIG thanks to all the people who so generously gave me feedback and/or helped me edit the book, including: Linda Hunter Adams, Laura Bridgewater, Debbie Christofferson, Christie Cosky, Jessica Duffett, Susan Eliason, Rebekah George, Cynthia Doxey Green, Julene Humes, Michael Hunter, Laura Jefferies, Orva Johnson, Joyce Kinmont, Jessica Knutson, Meldon Larson, Laura Lawrence, Stan and Sharon Miller, David Moore, Russ Osguthorpe, Mavis Parkinson, Steve Peck, Michael Sanders, Chantel Sloan, Alan Wilkins, Christina Williams, and Cynthia Wong. There were many others who made useful comments or gave me encouragement—thank you all!

Doug Heatherly (lighthouse24.com) was very patient in answering the many questions I sent him about the publishing process. Thanks, Doug!

Last, thanks to Dustin Schwanger for the beautiful typesetting and helping me to get it right. And to my partner in creating the cover, Bronson Terry: xie xie ni!

# Notes

ഗ

## Chapter 1 – Awakening to the Word of Wisdom

1. My experience is not shared by all who adopt this diet. I've since discovered that learning to cook and enjoy this food is not necessarily a major obstacle. Many people enjoy the food from the start, and everyone seems to love it before too long.

2. T. Colin Campbell and Thomas M. Campbell II, *The China Study: The Most Comprehensive Study of Nutrition Ever Conducted and the Startling Implications for Diet, Weight Loss, and Long-term Health* (Dallas: Benbella, 2006).

## Chapter 2 – The Flesh of Beasts

1. *Webster's Dictionary* (1828), s.v. "sparingly," http://machaut.uchicago.edu/websters. All further references to Webster's 1828 Dictionary come from this site.

2. This is based on research I've done on D&C 89:13 by analyzing the literature on the Word of Wisdom from 1833 to 2013. My conclusions are summarized in two manuscripts (submitted for publication in 2013): "Questioning the Comma in the Word of Wisdom" and "Getting into the Meat of the Word of Wisdom."

3. Harold McGee, *On Food and Cooking: The Science and Lore of the Kitchen* (New York: Charles Scribner's Sons, 1984), 123.

4. Vitamin D requires sunlight, and Vitamin B12 is made by bacteria. B12 is found in most animal foods (from the bacteria in the gut of the animal), but it is largely absent from our plant foods, partly due to modern sanitation. Current science suggests that people who abstain from all animal foods should take a B12 supplement. People who do not get enough sunlight to produce enough Vitamin D may also consider taking a Vitamin D supplement.

5. T. Colin Campbell, *Whole: Rethinking the Science of Nutrition* (New York: Ben-Bella Books, 2013), 254.

6. Alona Pulde and Matthew Lederman, *Keep It Simple, Keep It Whole: Your Guide to Optimum Health* (Los Angeles: Exsalus Health & Wellness Center, 2009). See chapter 8, "Protein" and chapter 11, "Fats and Oils."

7. Unfortunately, fish is not a healthier form of animal flesh. Fish generally have all the same drawbacks as any other form of flesh, and they are often much higher in contaminants. See, for example, John A. McDougall, "Fish is Not Health Food," (February 2003), http://www.nealhendrickson.com/mcdougall/030200pufishisnothealthfood.htm. Some fish is higher in omega 3, but we can get the omega 3 we need from plants, without the cholesterol, saturated fat, and contaminants.

8. You can test the amount of amino acids (along with fats and carbohydrates) in foods yourself using the handy nutrition calculator at http://cronometer.com.

9. Campbell and Campbell, *The China Study*, chapter 3.

10. Compare, for example, the China described by Campbell in *The China Study* with the chronic exposion of diabetes described by Yu Xu, et al. in "Prevalence and Control of Diabetes in Chinese Adults" (*Journal of the American Medical Association* 30, no. 9 (September 4, 2013): 948-958. China now has one of the highest rates of diabetes in the world.

11. *Handbook 2: Administering the Church*, Section 21.3.11, "Word of Wisdom" (Salt Lake City: The Church of Jesus Christ of Latter-day Saints, 2010).

# Chapter 3 – Wholesome Herbs and Every Fruit

1. See "Jamieson-Fausset-Brown Bible Commentary" on Daniel 1:12, http://biblehub.com/daniel/1-12.htm (accessed July 6, 2013).

2. Kim O'Neill and Byron Murray, *Power Plants: New Evidence That Natures Phytofighters Are Your Best Medicine* (Pleasant Grove, UT: Woodland, 2002).

3. To better understand the amazing complexity and power of plants, I recommend Colin Campbell's *Whole* and Joel Fuhrman, *Eat to Live: The Amazing Nutrient-Rich Program for Fast and Sustained Weight Loss* (New York: Little, Brown and Company, 2003).

4. See Campbell, *Whole*, and John A. McDougall, *The Starch Solution* (New York: Rodale, 2012).

5. Michael Pollan, *Food Rules: An Eater's Manual* (New York: Penguin Books), 29.

6. Fuhrman, *Eat to Live*, chapter 2.

7. Jeff Novick, "A Date With Disaster: The Pleasure Trap of Whole Natural Foods" (June 27, 2012), http://www.jeffnovick.com/RD/Articles/Entries/2012/6/27_A_Date_With_Disaster_The_Pleasure_Trap_of_Whole_Natural_Foods.html.

8. Joseph Fielding Smith, "The Word of Wisdom," *Improvement Era* (February 1956): 78–79.

9. Body K. Packer, "The Word of Wisdom: The Principle and the Promises," *Ensign* (April 1996): 17.

10. LDS Newsroom, "Mormonism in the News: Getting It Right," August 28, 2012, http://www.mormonnewsroom.org/article/mormonism-news--getting-it-right-august-29.

11. Coconut oil may not be the worst form of fat, but I believe the evidence does not support it as a "health food." Even assuming it is true that the medium-chain fatty acids (MCFAs) coconut oil contains are better health-wise then the long-chain fatty acids, about 40% of the saturated fat in coconut oil is not MCFAs. In fact, coconut oil contains almost as much long-chain saturated fat (35%) as lard (40%) (see the National Nutrient Database). The miniscule amount of nutrients there is in coconut oil can be found in rich abundance in whole-plant foods, without all the saturated fat, not to mention the calories.

12. Pulde and Lederman, *Keep It Simple, Keep It Whole.* See chapter 11, "Fats and Oils." They quote the National Academy of Sciences which has determined that an "adequate daily intake of omega-3 fatty acids is 1.1 grams for women and 1.6 grams for men." This amount equals about 1/4 to 1/3 of a teaspoon a day (p. 87). They also note that the unbalanced ratio of omega 6 to omega 3 fats in vegetable oils can be detrimental to our bodies because these two essential fats compete for the same enzymes.

13. Caldwell B. Esselstyn, Jr., *Prevent and Reverse Heart Disease* (New York: Avery, 2007), 85.

# Chapter 4 – All Grain is Good

1. *Merriam-Webster Online Dictionary* (2013), http://www.merriam-webster.com/dictionary/staple.

2. John A. McDougall, "Excerpt from *The Starch Solution*," February 2012, http://www.drmcdougall.com/misc/2012nl/feb/excerpt.htm.

3. John A. McDougall, "Introduction to New McDougall Book—*The Starch Solution*," February 2009, http://www.drmcdougall.com/misc/2009nl/feb/starch.htm.

4. McGee, *On Food and Cooking*, 226.

5. McGee, *On Food and Cooking*, 226–227.

6. Most low-carb and Paleo proponents (along with some high profile vegetarians) are strongly anti-grain. The books *Wheat Belly* by William Davis and *Grain Brain* by David Perlmutter are just two recent examples. According to Davis, "Wheat is the most destructive thing you could put on your plate, no question." (http://www.npr.org/blogs/thesalt/2013/09/26/226510988/doctors-say-changes-in-wheat-do-not-explain-rise-of-celiac-disease)

7. McDougall, *The Starch Solution*, 6–10.

8. Rob Dunn, "Human Ancestors Were Nearly All Vegetarians," *Scientific American*, July 23, 2012, http://blogs.scientificamerican.com/guest-blog/2012/07/23/human-ancestors-were-nearly-all-vegetarians.

9. Campbell and Campbell's *The China Study* is one excellent example. Though the work done in China is just one feature of the book, that work is the most comprehensive study of nutrition ever conducted.

10. Yu Xu, et al., "Prevalence and Control of Diabetes in Chinese Adults," *Journal of the American Medical Association* 30, no. 9 (September 4, 2013): 948–958.

11. National Diabetes Information Clearinghouse, "Obesity Associated with High Rates of Diabetes in the Pima Indians," in *Pima Indians: Pastfinders for Heath* (May 2002), http://diabetes.niddk.nih.gov/dm/pubs/pima/obesity/obesity.htm.

12. McDougall, *The Starch Solution*, chapter 1.

13. Lester E. Bush Jr., "The Word of Wisdom in Early Nineteenth-Century Perspective," *Dialogue* 14, no. 3 (Autumn 1981): 59.

14. Vermont Department of Health, "An Overview of Chronic Disease in Vermont," 2011, http://healthvermont.gov/research/chronic/overview.aspx.

15. Campbell and Campbell, *The China Study*, 191.

16. Editorial, *The Lancet* 378, no. 9790 (August 6, 2011): 457.

17. World Health Organization (WHO), "Noncommunicable Diseases Fact Sheet," (March 2013), http://www.who.int/mediacentre/factsheets/fs355/en.

18. Jared Diamond, *Guns, Germs, and Steel: The Fate of Human Societies* (New York: W. W. Norton & Company, 1997).

19. Richard Knox, "How Using Antibiotics In Animal Feed Creates Superbugs." NPR *The Salt*, February 21, 2012, http://www.npr.org/blogs/thesalt/2012/02/21/147190101/how-using-antibiotics-in-animal-feed-creates-superbugs). See also David Schardt, "Antibiotic Resistance: Wasting a Precious Saver." *Nutrition Action Healthletter*, (May 2013): 9–11 [http://www.cspinet.org/nah/pdfs/article-ABR.pdf].

20. "Talking Turkey: Our New Tests Show Reasons for Concern," *Consumer Reports* (June 2013): 46 [entire article, pp. 46–48].

21. Gardiner Harris, "Administration Seeks to Restrict Antibiotics in Livestock." *The New York Times*, July 13, 2009, http://www.nytimes.com/2009/07/14/health/policy/14fda.html.

22. World Health Organization (WHO), "Drug-resistant tuberculosis now at record levels," (March 2010), http://www.who.int/mediacentre/news/releases/2010/drug_resistant_tb_20100318.

23. Center for Disease and Control Prevention (CDC), "Antibiotic Resistance Threats in the United States, 2013," (April 2013), http://www.cdc.gov/drugresistance/threat-report-2013.

24. Todd Sperry, "New Push to Reduce Antibiotic Use in Farm Animals," CNN, September 23, 2012, http://www.cnn.com/2012/09/19/politics/antibiotic-use.

25. Spencer W. Kimball, "Why Call Me Lord, Lord, and Do Not the Things Which I Say?" *Ensign* (May 1975): 4.

# Chapter 5 – What about Dairy and Eggs?

1. John A. McDougall, *The McDougall Program for a Healthy Heart* (New York: Plume, 1996), 13–14.

2. Joseph Keon, *Whitewash: The Disturbing Truth about Cow's Milk and Your Health* (Gabriola Island, Canada: New Society Publishers, 2010). This is one of the most detailed resources on dairy.

3. Campbell, *Whole*, 39. See also Campbell and Campbell, *The China Study*.

4. Keon, *Whitewash*, 45.

5. Campbell and Campbell, *The China Study*, beginning on page 304, offers a good discussion of this topic. A more in-depth analysis is in Keon's *Whitewash*.

6. Amy Joy Lanou, "Should Dairy Be Recommended as Part of a Healthy Vegetarian Diet? Counterpoint," *American Journal of Clinical Nutrition*, 89, no. 5 (May 2009): 1638S–1642S. See also Keon, *Whitewash*, pp. 166–171 and "Preventing and Reversing Osteoporosis," Physicians Committee for Responsible Medicine, (accessed November 3, 2012), http://offices.ext.vt.edu/carroll/programs/anr/farm_management/cow_herd_performance.pdf.

7. Keon, *Whitewash*, 171–179. See also Brenda Davis and Vesanto Melina, *Becoming Vegan: The Complete Guide to Adopting a Healthy Plant-Based Diet* (Summertown, Tennessee: Book Publishing Company, 2000).

8. John A. McDougall, "When Friends Ask: 'Why Don't You Drink Milk?'" March 2007, http://drmcdougall.com/misc/2007nl/mar/dairy.htm.

9. Scott P. Greiner, "Cow Herd Performance and Profitability: Measuring How You Stack Up," Virginia Cooperative Extension, March 29, 2010, http://offices.ext.vt.edu/carroll/programs/anr/farm_management/cow_herd_performance.pdf.

10. Gordon B. Hinckley, "The Scourge of Illicit Drugs," *Ensign* (November 1989), 50.

# Chapter 6 – Science and the Word of Wisdom

1. Ali H. Mokdad, James S. Marks, Donna F. Stroup, and Julie L. Gerberding, "Actual Causes of Death in the United States, 2000," *Journal of the American Medical Association* 291, no. 10 (2004): 1238–1245.

2. Colin Spencer, *Vegetarianism: A History* (London: Grub Street, 2000), chapters 2–4.

3. Spencer, *Vegetarianism*, chapters 5–7.

4. John A. Widtsoe and Leah D. Widtsoe, *The Word of Wisdom, a Modern Interpretation* (Salt Lake City: Deseret Book, 1937) [http://discoveringthewordofwisdom.com/widtsoe-word-of-wisdom-1937].

5. American Dietetic Association, "Position of the American Dietetic Association: Vegetarian Diets," 2009, http://www.vrg.org/nutrition/2009_ADA_position_paper.pdf.

6. John A. Widtsoe and Leah D. Widtsoe, *The Word of Wisdom, a Modern Interpretation* (Salt Lake City: Deseret News Press, 1950).

7. Ray G. Cowley, MD, "An 1833 Guide for the Prevention of Heart Disease," *Improvement Era* (August, 1969): 60–63.

8. Gordon B. Hinckley, "Living Worthy of the Girl You Will Someday Marry," *Ensign* (May 1998): 49–51.

9. Kenneth E. Johnson, MD, *The Word of Wisdom Food Plan: A Medical Review of the Mormon Doctrine* (Springville, UT: Cedar Fort, 1993). See also Earl F. Updike, *The Mormon Diet—A Word of Wisdom: 14 Days to New Vigor and Health* (Bayfield, Colorado: Best Possible Health, 1991). Earl Updike and Kenneth Johnson were close friends. They both took a whole food, plant-based approach to the Word of Wisdom, so their books are forerunners to this book.

10. Bush, "The Word of Wisdom." The entire article speaks to this point.

11. Bush, "Word of Wisdom."

12. Joseph Smith, *Teachings of the Prophet Joseph Smith 1842–1843* (Salt Lake City: Deseret Book, 1938), 256.

13. Dan Buettner, *The Blue Zones: Lessons for Living Longer from the People Who've Lived the Longest* (Washington D.C.: National Geographic, 2008).

14. Institute of Church Ministry, " General Conference of Seventh-day Adventists: Three Strategic Issues, A World Survey." A Report Prepared for the Strategic Planning Commission. Seventh-day Adventist Theological Seminary, Andrews University, October 7, 2002. (See question 26).

15. Hugh Nibley, "Word of Wisdom: Commentary on D&C 89," 1979, [http://publications.maxwellinstitute.byu.edu/fullscreen/?pub=1044&index=1].

# Chapter 7 – Common Objections

1. Michael Pollan, *The Omnivore's Dilemma: A Natural History of Four Meals* (New York: Penguin Books), 96.

2. For an excellent discussion of the impact of industry on the nutritional advice to which Americans are exposed, see Campbell, *Whole.*

3. "Food & Addiction," *Nutrition Action Healthletter* (May 2012): 3–7 [http://www.drpeeke.com/data/images/nutrition_action_may_2012.pdf].

4. Douglas J. Lisle and Alan Goldhamer, *The Pleasure Trap: Mastering the Hidden Force That Undermines Health & Happiness* (Summertown, TN: Healthy Living, 2003), 22. See also the entire book (*The Pleasure Trap*), along with Neal D. Barnard, *Breaking the Food Seduction: The Hidden Reasons behind Food Cravings—And 7 Steps to End Them Naturally* (New York: St. Martin's Griffin, 2003).

5. Lisle and Goldhamer, *The Pleasure Trap*, chapter 7.

6. David A. Kessler, *The End of Overeating: Taking Control of the Insatiable American Appetite* (New York: Rodale, 2009).

7. This is particularly true of the Paleo community. See authors such as Loren Cordain, Mark Sisson, Robb Wolf, Art DeVany, and Boyd Eaton.

8. See authors such as Robert Atkins, Michael Eades, Mary Eades, Sally Fallon, Steve Phinney, Jeff Volek, Eric Westman, and Gary Taubes.

9. See authors such as Victoria Boutenko, David Wolfe, Douglas Graham, Paul Nison, and Natalia Rose. Some well-known raw food proponents are coming to recognize some drawbacks to a 100% raw diet and have backed down from an all-raw diet after years of claiming that anything but raw food is harmful to our bodies. See Victoria Boutenko, Elaina Love, and Chad Sarno, *Raw and Beyond: How Omega-3 Nutrition Is Transforming the Raw Food Paradigm* (Berkeley, CA: North Atlantic Books, 2012).

10. Like vegetable oils, nuts and seeds tend to have an unhealthy balance of omega 6 to omega 3 fats. For a balanced perspective on nuts, see: John A. McDougall, "Nuts Come in Hard Shells—for Reasons," November, 2009, http://www.drmcdougall.com/misc/2009nl/nov/nuts.htm. See also Jeff Novick, "Can't Lose The Weight? It Could Be The Nuts," July 26, 2012, http://www.vegsource.com/news/2012/07/cant-lose-the-weight-it-could-be-the-nuts.html.

11. Colin Campbell explores the impact of reductionist thinking on our understanding of nutrition in detail in his 2013 book, *Whole*. Our bodies are complex holistic organisms that depend on the complex holistic benefits of consuming whole foods, foods that contain all the complexity that God and nature designed them to contain. The prejudice of modern science is to reduce the complexity of human health to a combination of single, isolated factors. This decidedly

un-holistic approach vastly over-simplifies health and nutrition and inevitably leads to what appears to be profoundly contradictory bits of knowledge. While reductionist research has an important role to play in understanding nutrition, its dominance at the cost of every other approach primarily benefits the powerful food processing, drug, and supplement makers at the expense of good nutritional advice and the health and well-being of nearly everyone who consumes food.

12. Michael Pollan, *In Defense of Food: An Eater's Manifesto* (New York: Penguin Books), 62.

13. Campbell, *Whole*, inside book jacket.

14. Colin Campbell discusses all these issues very well in *Whole*.

15. Damien G. Finniss, Ted J. Kaptchuk, Franklin Miller and Fabrizio Benedetti, "Biological, Clinical, and Ethical Advances of Placebo Effects," *Lancet* 375, no. 9715 (February 20, 2010): 686–95.

16. Bruce H. Lipton, *The Biology of Belief: Unleashing the Power of Consciousness, Matter, & Miracles* (Philadelphia: Temple University Press, 2002).

17. Campbell, *Whole*, 151.

18. Years of consuming substances damaging to our bodies may contribute to gluten intolerance. This includes animal foods (especially animal protein), non-steroidal anti-inflammatory drugs (NSAIDs), and antibiotics. Eliminating these substances, along with gluten and foods that are causing problems, can help the body to heal and may lead to being able to tolerate whole plant foods that were previously problematic. See John A. McDougall, "Allergic Reactions to Food," https://www.drmcdougall.com/health/education/health-science/common-health-problems/allergic-reactions-to-food/ and "Diet: Only Hope for Arthritis," www.drmcdougall.com/health/education/health-science/featured-articles/articles/diet-only-hope-for-arthritis/; chapters 11 and 12 in Kirk Hamilton, *Staying Healthy in the Fast Lane: 9 Simple Steps to Optimal Health* (Sacramento: Prescription 2000, Inc.); and chapter 2 in Vesanto Melina, Jo Stepaniak, and Dina Aronson, *Food Allergy: Survival Guide* (Summertown Tennessee, Healthy Living Publications).

19. I am indebted to Dr. John McDougall for this thought.

20. Esselstyn, *Prevent and Reverse Heart Disease,* and Campbell and Campbell, *The China Study.*

21. Fuhrman, *Eat to Live*, 49.

22. Gladys Block, "Foods Contributing to Energy Intake in the US: Data from NHANES III and NHANES 1999–2000," *Journal of Food Composition and Analysis* 17 (2004): 442.

# Chapter 8 – Stewards of the Earth

1. 1 Timothy 4:3 is often cited as evidence for the case against abstaining from meat. In this chapter, Paul speaks of heresies in the last days, specifically, "Forbidding to marry, and commanding to abstain from meats, which God hath created to be received with thanksgiving of them which believe and know the truth" (1 Timothy 4:3). Note that the Greek word for *meats* in this verse means "whatever is eaten," or in other words, *food*. Most translations use the phrase *certain foods* instead of *meats* in this verse (see http://biblehub.com/1_timothy/4-3.htm), though the word in this context may have referred more specifically to animal flesh. The King James translators used the word *meat* because this word *meat* meant "food" for much of the English language history. Consider this verse in Genesis: "And God said, Behold, I have given you every herb bearing seed, which is upon the face of all the earth, and every tree, in the which is the fruit of a tree yielding seed; to you it shall be for meat" (Genesis 1:29). Note also that the word "meats" in D&C 49:18 may also mean "food." In verse 19, God explains *meats* to include not just beasts and fowls but also "that which cometh of the earth," or in other words, plants (D&C 49:19).

2. Steven C. Harper, *Setting the Record Straight: The Word of Wisdom* (Orem, UT: Millennial Press, 2007), 23.

3. For an excellent exploration of the meaning of "dominion," see Hugh Nibley, *Brother Brigham Challenges the Saints* (Salt Lake City: Deseret Book, 1994), chapter 1, "Man's Dominion, or Subduing the Earth."

4. Nibley, "Word of Wisdom."

5. Nibley, *Brother Brigham Challenges the Saints*, chapter 2, "Brigham Young on the Environment."

6. John Robbins, *The Food Revolution: How Your Diet Can Help Save Your Life and Our World* (San Francisco: Conari Press, 2001). See also: John Robbins, *Diet for a New America: How Your Food Choices Affect Your Health, Happiness and the Future of Life on Earth* (New York: Avon, 1992).

7. See, for example, "Meat.Org," PETA, 2012, http://www.meat.org.

8. David Pimentel and Marcia Pimentel, "Sustainability of Meat-based and Plant-based Diets and the Environment," *American Journal of Clinical Nutrition* 78(suppl) (2003): 660S–3S.

9. See estimates in Robbins, *The Food Revolution*, 236–237.

10. Robbins, *The Food Revolution*, chapter 15.

11. "Health Implications of Global Warming: Impacts on Vulnerable Populations," Physicians for Social Responsibility, http://www.psr.org/assets/pdfs/vulnerable-populations.pdf (accessed November 3, 2012).

12. Henning Steinfeld, et al., *Livestock's Long Shadow: Environmental Issues and Options* (Rome: United Nations Food and Agricultural Organization, 2006), http://www.fao.org/docrep/010/a0701e/a0701e00.htm.

13. Gidon Eshel and Pamela A. Martin, "Diet, Energy, and Global Warming." *Earth Interactions* 10, no. 9 (2005).

14. Elke Stehfest, et al., "Climate Benefits of Changing Diet," *Climatic Change* 95 (2009): 83–102.

15. Harold J. Marlow, et al., "Diet and the Environment: Does What You Eat Matter?" *American Journal of Clinical Nutrition* 89(suppl) (2009): 1699S–703S.

16. United Nations, "Livestock's Long Shadow."

17. Robbins, *The Food Revolution*, 241.

18. Bill McKibben, "The Only Way to Have a Cow," *Orion Magazine* (March/April 2010), https://orionmagazine.org/article/the-only-way-to-have-a-cow/.

19. Philip Wollen, "Philip Wollen, Australian Philanthropist, Former VP of Citibank, Makes Blazing Animal Rights Speech," (June 24, 2012), http://freefromharm.org/videos/educational-inspiring-talks/philip-wollen-australian-philanthropist-former-vp-of-citibank-makes-blazing-animal-rights-speech.

20. Brigham Young, "Weakness and Impotence of Men—Condition of the Saints—Dedication to the Lord—The Millennium" (April 6, 1852), transcribed by G. D. Watt. *Journal of Discourses* 1, no. 31(1853–1886): 198–203.

21. Gerald E. Jones, *Concern for Animals as Manifest in Five American Churches: Bible Christian, Shaker, Latter-day Saint, Christian Scientist and Seventh-Day Adventist* (PhD diss., Brigham Young University, 1972).

22. Joseph Smith, *Documentary History of the Church*, vol. 2 (Salt Lake City: Deseret News, 1904), 71–72.

23. George Q. Cannon, "Wanton Killing," *Juvenile Instructor* 24, no. 23 (December 1, 1889): 548–549.

24. Jones, *Concern for Animals*, 58.

25. Heber C. Kimball, in *Journal of Discourses* 5, no. 137 (August 2, 1857).

26. Horne, *Journals of Abraham H. Cannon*, 424.

27. Joseph Fielding Smith, "Is It a Sin to Kill Animals Wantonly?" *Improvement Era* (August 1961): 568.

28. Johnson, *The Word of Wisdom Food Plan*, 18.

29. Joseph F. Smith, "Humane Day," *Juvenile Instructor* 53 no. 4 (April 1918): 182–183.

# Chapter 9 – Why Doesn't the Church Tell Us?

1. Heber J. Grant, *The Millennial Star* 57, no. 7 (February 14, 1895): 101.

2. Paul Y. Hoskisson, "The Word of Wisdom in Its First Decade," *Journal of Mormon History* 38, no. 1 (2012): 131–200.

3. Paul H. Peterson, *An Historical Analysis of the Word of Wisdom* (M.A. thesis, Brigham Young University, August 1972). Note: I rely on Peterson's excellent thesis for background history throughout this entire section.

4. Leonard J. Arrington, "An Economic Interpretation of the 'Word of Wisdom.'" *Brigham Young University Studies* 1, no. 1 (Winter 1959): 37–49.

5. Quoted in Peterson, *An Historical Analysis of the Word of Wisdom*, 66.

6. Heber J. Grant, *The Millennial Star* 57, no. 7 (February 14, 1895): 97–98.

7. Quoted in Peterson, *An Historical Analysis of the Word of Wisdom*, 97.

8. Peterson, *An Historical Analysis of the Word of Wisdom*, 90.

9. Richard Cowan, *Doctrine & Covenants: Our Modern Scripture* (Provo, UT: Brigham Young University Press, 1978).

10. *History of the Church*, 6:184–85; from a discourse given by Joseph Smith on Jan. 21, 1844, in Nauvoo, Illinois; reported by Wilford Woodruff.

11. George A. Smith, "Gathering and Sanctification of the People of God." March 18, 1855. *Reported By: G. D. Watt.*

12. Smith, "Gathering and Sanctification of the People of God."

13. See chapter 8, note 1.

14. Quoted in Peterson, *An Historical Analysis of the Word of Wisdom*, 96–97.

15. Rick B. Jorgensen, *Not by Commandment or Constraint: The Relationship between the Dietary Behaviors of College-Aged Latter-day Saints and Their Interpretation of the Word of Wisdom"* (PhD diss., Brigham Young University, August 2008).

16. Lester E. Bush, Jr. *Health and Medicine among the Latter-day Saints* (New York: Crossroad, 1993), 67.

17. Ray M. Merrill and Steven Hillam, "Religion and Body Weight in Utah," *Utah's Health: An Annual Review* 11 (2006): 40–50.

18. You can find several examples on the Church's website (http://www.lds.org). Type the following into the search box, including the quote marks: "word of wisdom" and vegetables.

19. Hyrum Smith, *Times and Seasons* 3, no. 15 (June 1, 1842): 799–801.

20. Church Historian's Office, *Journal History of the Church (*March 11, 1897): 2.

21. Church Historian's Office, *Journal History of the Church* (May 5, 1898): 2–3.

22. Joseph F. Merrill, *Conference Report* (Salt Lake City: The Church of Jesus Christ of Latter-day Saints, April 1948): 70–75.

23. Ezra Taft Benson, "In His Steps," BYU Devotional (1979), https://speeches.byu.edu/talks/ezra-taft-benson_in-christs-steps/.

24. Gordon B. Hinckley, "Mormon Should Mean 'More Good,'" *Ensign* (November 1990): 51.

25. Gordon B. Hinckley, "My Testimony," *Ensign* (November 1993): 51.

26. Heber J. Grant, *LDS Annual Conference Report* (Salt Lake City: The Church of Jesus Christ of Latter-day Saints, April 1937), 15.

27. Robert Murray Stewart, "A Normal Day in the Home of George Albert Smith," *Improvement Era* (April, 1950): 287.

28. Jones, *Concern for Animals*, 115–118.

29. "Jessie Evans Smith's Ninety-Minute Bread," *Improvement Era* (April 1970): 59.

30. Paul H. Peterson, "The Sanctity of Food: A Latter-day Saint Perspective," in *Religious Educator* 2, no. 1 (Provo, UT: BYU Religious Studies Center, 2001), 41.

31. Spencer W. Kimball, "Strengthening the Family—the Basic Unit of the Church," *Ensign* (May 1978).

32. Spencer W. Kimball, "Fundamental Principles to Ponder and Live," LDS General Conference (October 1978).

# Chapter 10 – The Promised Blessings

1. Harold B. Lee, *The Teachings of Harold B. Lee* (Salt Lake City: Desert Book, 1996), 205.

2. George Q. Cannon, "Topic of the Times," *Juvenile Instructor* 27, no. 22 (November 15, 1892): 689–691.

3. Stephen L Richards, "Keep the Commandments," In *LDS Conference Report* (April 1949): 141.

4. Russell M. Nelson, "Decisions for Eternity," LDS General Conference (October 2013).

5. Boyd K. Packer, "Revelation in a Changing World," LDS General Conference (October 1989).

6. Peterson, "The Sanctity of Food."

7. Thomas G. Alexander, *Mormonism in Transition* (Chicago: University of Illinois, 1986), 270.

# Index

# Y

## Scriptural References

*Entries which include (JST) indicate that the citation is taken from the Joseph Smith translation of the Bible.*

26781108R00130

Made in the USA
Columbia, SC
12 September 2018